Testosterone Replacement Therapy

One Man's Journey To A Better Life

Rowdy Rawson

Book cover design by Rebecacovers

ISBN: 978-0-578-52177-0

Bearface Publishing
P.O. Box 93
Iuka, MS 38852
www.mytrtjourney.com

CONTENTS

DISCLAMER

I am not your doctor! The content of this book is not intended to be a substitute for professional medical advice, diagnosis, or treatment. Always seek the advice of your physician or other qualified health provider with any questions you may have regarding a medical condition.

INTRODUCTION

I am happy to be sharing the following account of my experience with testosterone replacement therapy, or TRT as I will refer to it through this book. I tried my best to record my overall mood, my experiences good and bad, and the changes in me both physically and mentally during my journey.

First, let me share a bit about who I am and how I ended up in a place to even consider TRT. I have been healthy pretty much all of my life. I have never been seriously overweight, although I always seemed to have to watch what I eat in order to avoid gaining weight. I have been active throughout adulthood. Lifting weights, jogging, golf, hiking. There was a period in my early 30's where I stopped being so active and I let my weight creep up on me, but even then I was just a little chubby and never seriously obese. When I divorced at 35, it was relatively easy to drop the weight through improved diet and exercise. In fact, by the time I hit 40 in 2015 I was possibly in the best shape of my life. I felt good. I looked good. Life was good. Until it wasn't.

In the fall of 2015 I began to notice a couple of odd things about myself. I began feeling a lot of stiffness in my joints, and my mood was fluctuating from high to low with no evident reason for either. I would have days where I just felt "off", and days where everything was just fine. A sort of fogginess settled in over my brain, and I began to have trouble concentrating. Then I got a bout of insomnia where I slept only hours per week. I would lie in bed at night tired but wired and drift off just before the sun came up, only to wake with a start covered in sweat. I dropped a good bit of weight and got down too light for my frame. I no longer looked or felt good.

Something was going haywire with my body and mind, and at the time I attributed it all to stress. Work was demanding. I had a bad break up with a girlfriend that summer. I was not getting along with my ex-wife, and I really hated the small town I seemed to be stuck in. About the only positive was the time spent with my daughter. I took a break from the gym and tried some things to relax more. Long Epsom salt baths, meditation, some herbal sleep remedies. Things got a little better. Winter came and my mood was sort of kind of stable. I had added some weight back, was sleeping okay, and the night sweats were subsiding.

But a pain developed in my right hip that was really troublesome. I thought at the time I had injured it doing squats at the gym, though I could not recall any particular workout where an injury occurred. I began going to a chiropractor and got temporary relief every other week or so. Then the pain spread to the other hip. No more squats for me. My mood began going up and down again, and at times I actually found myself crying while driving home. For no reason at all. A childhood memory would flash across my mind or a song from my youth would come on the radio and it would be Niagara Falls. Little triggers that would send me into a sobbing fit. I was losing it, man. Then my shoulders began really hurting. Both of them. Again, I attributed this to something I was doing wrong in the gym. No more pressing exercises. My neck stiffened up. My knees began to ache. My elbows hurt. I began to get really scared. But, being the stubborn jackass of a man I was at the time I did not seek medical care. I continued my chiropractic treatments and Epsom baths, I slept when I could, tried to cut back my travel for work and do more from the home office, until finally something happened that was just not acceptable.

In April of 2016, I attended a concert with a female friend and forced myself to have a good time in spite of my deteriorating condition. I had a few beers and about 8 ibuprofen, we had some laughs, and eventually made it back to our hotel room. I was ready for action even if I felt crappy. But things went south quickly. This girl was hot with fake breasts and a spectacular body. But my downstairs buddy just could not rise to the occasion. This was a disaster of epic proportions. I was mentally broken. I slept fitfully, watching the silhouette of a beautiful woman lay in disappointment beside me. I vowed to get this shit fixed whatever in the hell it was.

The next week I went to the doctor finally. I saw a nurse practitioner at the local clinic, and brought a list of my symptoms as they were so long by this point. Below is the list I took with me and rattled off to the amazement of the young Nurse Practitioner.

Muscle loss/weakness
Weight gain
Sore throat
Difficulty swallowing
Fatigue
Frequent urination
Loss of hair on legs
ED
Nails thickening
Dry skin
Dandruff
Brain fog
Severe hip and shoulder pain
Right thumb pain
Back pain
Left jaw pain
Neck pain
Knee pain
Dark circles under eyes
Depression
Anxiety
Cold hands and feet
Poor circulation in hands
Night sweats

She stopped writing about half way through and said, "we need to start drawing blood now." They took a bunch of blood from me and scheduled a follow up in a few days. She prescribed some Meloxicam which is an anti-inflammatory, and I hobbled out of there relieved to finally get some answers.

I went back a few days later to follow up her and was told the following.

"You likely have either lupus or rheumatoid arthritis, or possible multiple sclerosis. You don't test exactly positive for any of them, but there are indicators. Your inflammation markers are extremely elevated which is a sign for immune issues, and all of your joint and muscle pain could fit with any of those. I am referring you to a specialist, but they cannot see you until early June." My heart sank. Any of those illnesses would require a lifelong battle and result in a shorter lifespan. And I was not sure I could make it another 6 weeks just to see a specialist. I felt like I was dying right then and there. I felt like I was fucked honestly.

I struggled through the remainder of spring and my health slid further downhill. My right knee begin to swell along with both ankles. I developed a rash on my legs, and it hurt to even move. I survived on high doses of Aleve and ibuprofen. At long last my appointment with the specialist came. My dad had to drive me to the visit.

The rheumatologist met with me and heard my story and said she did not actually think I had any of the aforementioned afflictions suggested by the Nurse Practitioner, but would draw some blood and run her own tests. This was a relief, but it if wasn't any of those then what the hell was it? I hobbled out of there with more questions than answers. It was to be 2 weeks until I saw her again. She gave me a shot of decadron before I left and said it would relieve all of the joint pain for a month or so. I was ecstatic with the thought of just a little bit of relief!

2 weeks seemed like 2 years, but my follow up day came and again my dad drove me to the appointment. The shot that should have lasted a month lasted a day at best. It barely touched whatever in the hell I had.

The specialist reviewed my labs with me and declared that I did not have rheumatoid arthritis or lupus or any other ailment she could detect or treat. She suggested I see an endocrinologist and check my hormones. Okay.

I quickly got a referral and only had to wait a couple of weeks to see one. She reviewed my history and previous blood work and told me she doubted it was hormone related but would do her own blood work and we would see. I came back a week later for the news. My thyroid numbers were not great but not bad. TSH of around 3. My testosterone was lowish around 300, with estradiol on the low end at 12. Not great numbers but nothing to explain the pain and other various symptoms I was experiencing. It could possibly explain the ED which was still there I was sure. I had not ventured out to have sex again since that night in the spring, but my morning erections were completely absent and I had no desire at all to have sex. We discussed possible treatment but agreed I really needed to figure out the source of this before I did anything else. Where to go next?

My ex-wife is a Nurse Practitioner, but I had never allowed her to treat me. She was aware of my ailment in general, although I hid most of the really bad stuff. I did not want to risk her using my health as a reason to begin a damn custody battle. We were getting along better but I did not fully trust her. I did trust her medical skills though, and I reviewed all of my findings so far with her. I had also been doing my own research on the internet of people with similar symptoms with difficulty getting a diagnosis, and I kept finding similar stories as mine with one culprit involved: Lyme disease.

I had never known anyone with this and always thought it was easy to treat if you got a tick bite. But what I found was if you don't catch it early it can be damned hard to eradicate and wreak havoc on the body. There were a couple of types of doctors who treat this: infectious disease specialists and what are known as Lyme Literate MDs. I opted for the first one since my ex-wife knew of one in the next town over.

She got me an appointment the following week and I again hobbled my broken ass into a doctor's waiting room and hoped I would find answers and help. The lady listened to my story and then told me, "I can tell you that you very likely have Lyme disease and need look no further for a diagnosis. But I can also tell you that treatment options are very limited and can often not perform any better than just allowing time to heal you. Which can take up to 10 years or more in some cases." I could not believe this! 10 years! No way would I last that long in this condition. She started my on doxycycline for 30 days and I was on my way.

I'd like to tell you that 30 days of antibiotics cleared everything right up, but it was only the beginning of my nightmare. I got worse before I saw some minor improvements, and I had to beg her for more of the doxycycline. I got 30 days more and then she cut me off and said she could offer no further treatment. My ex got me a little more doxy, but honestly it was not helping anymore. I was sinking fast. Depression. Anxiety beyond belief. Sex was an afterthought. I don't know if I could have had sex then and I did not care. No more gym. I worked from home and travelled for work when I had to, suffering alone in hotel rooms and trying not to overdose on ibuprofen. It was misery.

I found a Lyme Literate MD, or LLMD about 2 hours away and got an appointment in early January of 2017. My mom drove me. I felt like dying the whole way over.

The doctor reviewed my file from all my previous visits, along with the list of current symptoms I had printed out so I would not forget them. My mind was so warped at this point I could barely think coherently. I forgot a lot of things on a daily basis. I had fallen into a deep depression. Anxiety was riding my ass day and night. He listened to my story and for the first time said the words I had longed to hear, "I can help you." I wanted to cry right there in this man's office. I think I actually did a little bit but those days are not so clear.

It wasn't easy, but I began to crawl out of the fog and back into life. I took a small pharmacy of drugs to combat the infection raging inside my body, and slowly the pain begin to fade. I could jog again then run. I could lift baby weights then heavier ones. I began to remember who I was. I continued to get better physically into the summer, but then seemed to hit a wall. Depression had been lingering for months and would not budge, even while taking Trintellix. I still had bouts of anxiety and had to take Klonopin to make it through the majority of my days. I was able to lift weights again but making little to no progress. And I began dating again but could not have sex without Viagra or Cialis, and sometimes even then it was not what it should be.

I had my hormones checked a couple of times throughout my recovery and they were not getting better. 290. 320. 300. I was stuck at the low end. And my free testosterone was low as well, which I would come to learn was the more important of the two numbers. I needed help. I needed a boost to finish getting my life back. Summer came and went and I was hesitant to take that step. I visited with a reputable wellness clinic in the next town over, and the male nurse practitioner had been on TRT for over 10 years. He loved it. He was lean and fit in his early 60s and all smiles. Yet the thought of needles in my arm or leg for the rest of my life seemed a bridge too far, even after all I had been through. I thought about it daily. I prayed about it. I journaled. Fall came and I was losing interest in women altogether. Sad that I had to rely on PEDs to perform, and no libido to drive me to get better. Work was suffering. I felt stuck in a job I no longer enjoyed. I was better but just existing. Something had to give. Something had to change.

This is my story of how I finished getting my life back.

WHAT HAVE I GOT MYSELF INTO?

10/12/17 Thursday Day 1

Today I made a huge decision. A life changing decision. I have elected to begin TRT, or testosterone replacement therapy. After the past few years and the amount of suffering I have endured, I am hoping this is the final piece to my health puzzle that allows me to live a full and enriched life. I have done the research. I have read the testimonials good and bad. I have asked all the questions. I don't have all the answers but I feel like I know what to expect and that I am prepared for any hiccups. The wellness clinic I am using is reputable and knowledgeable. Everything is in place. Depression and fatigue are a bitch, and I have nowhere to go but up. Time to rock and roll.

I got my prescription filled this afternoon and a bag full of needles. I am all set. I now have a bottle of testosterone cypionate and a bottle of Pregnyl. Will it make me pregnant? Because I'll be pissed if that happens. Shit.

Before my first injection, I set my needles out and used the big one to deliver the solvent to the powder inside the Pregnyl bottle. It immediately dissolved and formed a clear liquid. Cool. I set it down and pulled up .5 mL of the testosterone into my syringe. The liquid was thick and took a bit to fill up the chamber. Once it hit the number I wiped a spot on my shoulder with an alcohol swab, depressed the needle until a drop came out the end, then sunk it in my left shoulder. It did not hurt at all. I could feel the liquid being absorbed and instantly got an erection. Just kidding.

Then the HCG. This liquid is not thick and easily drew into the syringe. I filled up .2 mL, squeezed the fat on my lower belly, and pushed it in. Did not hurt at all.

I took a minute to clean up my mess, and then I was done. Total time about 3 minutes. Not bad for the first day. I'll do this again Monday morning, keeping with my every 3.5 day schedule. I did a self-assessment to see if I felt like whipping somebody's ass, but I seem content to give everyone a pass today. So far so good.

10/13/17 Friday Day 2
It's Friday the 13th. A good omen. I am off work today and headed south to Gulf Shores, AL for the Shrimp Festival. I slept well last night. My daughter Scarlett and I went to the county fair and it was fun. I have a nice sense of calm this morning. Nothing outrageously different, but definitely a bit calmer. It's nice. Placebo effect? We will see.

I picked my buddy Jimmy up in Birmingham and we debated drinking beer on the way down. Not a good idea. I elected to wait until we were close which was the right move. Plenty of time for beer now that we are here. We talked on the way down mostly about women and money. I'd like to have more of each. He is married so I don't think he cares about either anymore. I would settle for some confidence and a clear mind at this point.

It's hot down here in Gulf Shores, and we worked on the condo all afternoon. Now we are taking a beer break and I am getting some quick writing done. Later we are going to the Shrimp Festival. I am hopeful, but for what I do not know.

11:11 PM It did not take long for that hope to be dashed as the festival turned out to be more like a county fair on the beach. The seafood was deep fried frozen for the most part. Definitely not local like I thought. These vendors seem to be from everywhere but Gulf Shores. Louisiana mostly. And there are hardly any pretty single ladies here. Lots of married ones. Plenty of heavy ones. But not many good looking single ones. Could I have talked to a cute woman? I don't think so. Not yet.

Later I called Steve, the taxi driver we always use when we are here. He picked us up in 15 minutes and shuttled us to the best bar on the Gulf Coast, the legendary Flora-Bama. It was wall to wall women and everyone was having a great time. We found a band in the back room called River Dan that is a young country boy playing solid gold outlaw country from the 1970's and 80's. It was an awesome night overall, and my mood was mostly positive. I did talk to a few girls, mostly just hi and how are you and what not. There was a blonde that I think wanted me to talk to her because she smiled and looked at me expectantly. I had no game and no confidence and let the moment pass. I still feel depressed but it is not overwhelming.

10/14/17 Saturday Day 3
I did not wake up with a raging erection like I thought I might this morning, but perhaps a night of drinking interfered with that. Maybe it takes a while before the T has any effect in that area. I look forward to having a youthful sex drive again. I feel like I lost a few years battling Lyme disease. Time to make up for it.

I am up at 9 AM getting ready to work the beer tent I volunteered for. I figured it would be a good way to meet people and force me to be sociable, but this was when I still thought the Shrimp Festival was cool. Now I'm thinking of skipping out, but I will honor my commitment and show up as scheduled.

In spite of the too many drinks I had last night, I don't feel bad at all. Not even tired. Maybe a bit dehydrated.

5:11 PM It was a nice day working the beer tent and I could see the ocean rolling in from where our tent was stationed. I still have a moderate feeling of wellbeing and it is still nice.

When my shift ended I discovered the next shift was comprised of 6 hot women. Figures. I was working with old dudes. I smiled at them and telepathically communicated my bad intentions, then I was on my way. I'm really dangerous right now.

Damn I feel better today. I decided to walk back to the condo since it was only a mile. It's hot but breezy down here on the Gulf.

This afternoon I sat peacefully in my beach chair and reflected on how at ease I feel. It's been so long since I could just enjoy any present moment. Lyme disease is hell. It is a disgrace that there is not an easy cure and the

CDC and Infectious Disease Society of America barely even acknowledge it is a problem. I've never even dreamed of suffering like that before. But I'm still here.

We talked about music and women and life. Our plans are to go back to the Flora-Bama and see River Dan again. One of the best bands I have seen in a long time. I am excited at the possibilities.

10/15/17 Sunday Day 4
Holy hell what happened? I feel like I got hit by a Mack truck. I can hear the traffic outside my condo window. It sounds like the vehicles are running through my head. My ears are ringing so loud that my head might burst. Jimmy is a dumbass. And I am even dumber. The clock says 11:21. I should already be on the road home.

We finished our work on the bunk bed and had lunch at Lou Lou's. There was a lively Sunday afternoon crowd and the couple of draft beers I had eased the pain of the hangover. We finally got on the road around 3:30 and I knew it would be a hellish drive home. I deserved what I got. Somehow, in spite of all that happened, I didn't feel *that* bad. Not as bad as I really should. When I first awoke it was rough, but once I got going everything seemed to settle down. I still have a sense of calm. A bit shakier but still overall calm. Nothing like the anxiety brought on by Lyme. That shit was awful.

On the way back we listened to The Game by Neil Strauss. It's about the underground world of pickup artists. Very entertaining. I debated with Jimmy learning these techniques at this point in my life. Why have I not told him about TRT? I tell him pretty much everything. But I never mentioned that all weekend. Maybe I wanted to see how this first month goes before I reveal anything? Should I be embarrassed? I don't think so. I do not really care what people think, least of all my best friend. I'll tell him eventually. I'll have to once I become little Hercules and women begin flocking to me. Ha.

We made it back to Birmingham in good time despite heavy traffic and rain. I realized on the way home that I cannot drink like that anymore. I don't want to drink like that anymore. I am committed to a clean diet and aggressive fitness regimen. I look forward to beginning to jog again. And I cannot wait to track my lifts in the gym and see some damn progress. How disheartening is has been to not be able to bust my ass in there and mostly lie around on the couch suffering these past few years. I am determined to make this a good thing.

10/16/17 Day 5
I woke up at 6:30 AM. I have to be in Jackson, TN for an audit. I slept about 6 hours and it appears to be enough. Another hour or two would have been nice but this is not bad. I remember the Lyme days where I could barely turn over to get my feet on the floor. I am thankful for these better days, but still I want more.

I already did my second round of shots. I set the testosterone and HCG out on the counter with my needles and alcohol and just stared at them for a minute. Am I really doing this? Some people mix them but I have not tried that. Maybe after I perfect this routine I'll look to refine it. I popped the testosterone in the same left deltoid. I should probably alternate. It hurt a bit this time. What changed? Karmic payback for abusing my body? The HCG hurt my belly fat as well. The old belly is definitely soft, but that will soon not be the case.

I felt okay on my drive to Jackson. Light anxiety. A bit of depression but I deserve it. Just some after effects of the copious amount of alcohol. I'll drink lots of water today to wash that out. It's odd how I can observe depression as a physical feeling rather than having sad thoughts about something. I never understood it before. I do now.

The audit went smoothly and I did good work at the plant. My job is not exciting but it is a good job and I enjoy it more than I used to. The work we do is important and helps keep people safe.

My headache from the teeth work I had done last week is finally gone. I was worried I might have a damn tumor the way it was radiating pain at times. But it has resolved itself. One thing I hope to gain from better testosterone and estrogen levels is less inflammation and less joint pain. After Lyme it would be nice to feel oiled up and fully lubricated.

Mentally the drive home was a bit foggy. I tried to talk myself into a good place but I am tired of talking myself into a good place. I never had to do that before. Hopefully the testosterone helps. I wanted to lift today but did not have time because Scarlett's mom will be dropping her off soon. I am determined to lift tomorrow and begin tracking my progress.

10/17/17 Tuesday Day 6
I woke up at 3:33 AM. Wide awake. I went to sleep at 10, so that is just over 5 hours of sleep. If I had known I would not go back to sleep then I would have gotten up and done something productive, but I assumed I would get sleepy and drift back off.

I did not have wood when I awoke and was disappointed. A funny thing happened later though. When I got up at 6 to get coffee going, old Mr. Wiggly sprung right up and greeted me. Weird. I guess that's something though.

My mind and vision were particularly clear this morning. Perhaps the brain fog is already beginning to lift. Emotionally I am optimistic about the day ahead. I like that. Too many mornings were spent waking up in a sea of pain and fog and just wanting to make it to bedtime. This is better.

I plan to call Kristi tonight. Some definite potential there. Odd that we would run into each other at a funeral and she would tell me that I looked good and to call her. Am I confident enough to call her?

The drive to Jackson was purposeful. I feel good about today. My boys are hanging a little high this morning. Not sure what is up with that but I am sure they will come down later. It was pretty chilly when I woke up.

As I walked around the plant finishing up my audit, I noticed that the friction of my pants caused me to become fully erect. That shit has not happened for a long time. This is a good sign of things to come. I want to call Kristi right now. What would I say?

I felt a little depression and no anxiety today. Brain fog was just enough to register, but overall in a better place. Derealization is still lingering, but I'm closer to reality than I was. I could get used to this. I hope it lasts.

This afternoon I held a close out meeting for the audit I conducted. It was me and 6 other men. Lots of ego in the room. I felt totally comfortable delivering the audit results to them and sitting around shooting the breeze afterwards. Sometimes I am not so comfortable in those situations, but today it felt natural.

At the gym this evening, I saw Katie whom I met when she worked at Piggly Wiggly. She is a tall, leggy, raven haired beauty and smiled and waved big when she saw me. Did she know something? Could she smell the testosterone? Nah, just being friendly. I chatted her up, and even though she is 15 years my junior, I felt like I had a chance with her. An odd feeling as my confidence with women has evaporated over the past few years. Do I have a chance? I'm still scared for some reason.

My workout was brief but intense. I focused on good form and really contracting the muscles as I pushed through. My shoulders feel good in spite of the pain from these past years. Better things are coming I hope. I see all these young meatheads throwing weight around and taking their hormonal youth for granted. Soon they will be wondering who the old dude is with the ripped physique. Soon.

We had dinner tonight for my sister's birthday. I was in a good mood and more talkative than usual. I solved the Wheel of Fortune puzzle before anyone else. Brain fog is definitely better. I ate steak and sweet potato, but skipped the cake and ice cream. I am dedicated to improving my mind and body. That caramel cake looked pretty damn good though.

I called Kristi tonight but she did not answer so I left a voicemail. I was kind of relieved she did not answer. Ridiculous at my age I know. I would like to have a date with her this weekend, but at the same time it frightens me. I have not dated a blonde in a long time, and even though I know she is not a true blonde it's the thought that counts.

10/18/17 Wednesday Day 7

I slept awesome last night. I felt a bit of anxiety around bedtime. Just a slight buzzing that was uncomfortable. It felt more Lyme related than anything else. That shit better not come back. I fell asleep around 10:15 and awoke in the middle of the night with a raging erection. I was so excited I almost got up to admire it in the mirror. But when I awoke again at 5AM it was gone. I had big plans of getting up super early to write and meditate and visualize. I hit the snooze a few times and got up at 6 feeling good but still no erection. No foggy brain and no soreness anywhere though. My boys are high and tight again this morning. It is cold again so maybe that is it? They had come back down yesterday after riding high most of the morning. Perhaps I should go play with them? Damn I need a woman.

I did a quick meditation and a super short visualization. Before Lyme I had just learned to use creative visualization to help accomplish my goals. I was getting some good results, but once I got sick it was too damned hard to picture anything worthy or feel good about anything other than wanting to feel good again. But I know it works so this morning's half-assed effort will have to get better. I'm still giving myself credit for waking up before dawn and getting my daughter ready for school early.

Feeling very focused this morning. Like today is a day I will get shit done. Working from home requires this kind of focus and it has not been here in a long time.

I was hungry this morning. I have been intermittent fasting off and on and usually do not eat breakfast, but I was genuinely hungry so I had some greek yogurt and a protein cookie. I feel better now but could eat some more. It will be advantageous to begin tracking calories. I'd hate to become a high T fatass.

I am also horny. It has been a month since I had sex. Even with low libido I need more sex than this. And I have not been masturbating which compounds the issue. I think I will go to the gym and do some cardio. Or masturbate. Or both.

2:01 PM. I did both. And enjoyed both.

Plenty of energy at the gym. I was going to ride the bike, but they got these new rowing machines and I wanted to try one. I did 2000 meters in less than 10 minutes and it was intense. I like that kind of workout. I certainly felt like I could do more.

I made an appointment with an acupuncturist to see about the ringing in my ears. He practices Chinese medicine so perhaps he can help with any remaining Lyme symptoms as well. Cool people those Chinese.

Mentally I am calm and focused today. Very little depression or anxiety. Derealization is mostly clear right now also. I watched my dog Chewy play in the backyard from the deck earlier and the world did not look like a 3D fun factory. Just trees and grass and a smartass little dog barking at squirrels. The way the world should be.

I knocked out 1000 words on my Lyme novel before I went to the gym. It took maybe 10 minutes, and it was good stuff. With this level of focus I'll have a rough draft by Christmas.

6:30 PM Scarlett is home and my head is hurting now. When she began bouncing a ball in the living room it annoyed me and I had to fight to keep from snapping at her. I need to eat something.

Kristi texted me back. She is travelling this week and won't be home until Saturday. I'll be at the MSU football game then and leaving Sunday to work in Ohio so no nookie for at least a week. Damnit. But she is definitely interested. Will I be able to pull it off? One can only hope. I am scared. Scared of pussy. Shit.

9:45 PM I felt better after eating and we watched some TV before bed.

Now that I am ready for sleep I feel keyed up. Insomnia better not come back. I hate that shit. A touch of anxiety just swept over me but it passed. What will life be like without anxiety if TRT helps?

10/19/17 Thursday Day 8
I woke up to the alarm at 5:45 and it wasn't happening. I was groggy and sleepy and felt a bit funky so I hit the snooze 6 times before finally getting up close to 7. I think I only got up to pee once last night though which is great. No morning wood today and that is disappointing.

I checked myself in the mirror expecting to see a full beard and huge biceps but saw neither. Just my soft belly and fuzzy goatee.

Once I got moving around I felt better but not as clear as yesterday. This evening it will be injection time. Have I been on this long enough to experience a trough? I don't think so. I got a semi-chubby walking to the kitchen so I guess that is better than nothing. I jotted down today's goals and objectives then woke Scarlett up for school. I had plans of going to the office this morning but elected to work from home instead. Sometimes being around a lot of people is hard to take. My left ear is ringing as usual as I write this. My boys were hanging low when I first awoke but drew up when I went outside to let Chewy out to pee. It was about 48 degrees this morning so I suppose they should have drawn up.

I was not hungry but elected to eat breakfast. Oatmeal with protein powder and almond milk. That's good, right? Seems like something a bodybuilder would eat.

After dropping Scarlett off I worked steadily until 11AM then got cleaned up to have lunch with Scarlett at her school. Will the teachers be able to resist themselves when I walk by smelling of testosterone? I'd hate to cause a scene. I know her gifted class teacher has the hots for me. If she pulls up her shirt when I walk by then I know to cut back my dosage.

1:16 PM Just got back from lunch. Nothing unusual happened. I did see the gifted teacher. We'll call her Dawn. When Dawn saw me walking by she came to an immediate halt and walked back toward me. Her smile was so big I thought she would devour me. She flirted a bit then shook it for me as she walked away. Does she want me? She wants me.

At the gym I had an intense workout. I was working back and biceps and doing some abs and felt good. I was able to squeeze out good sets and had energy for more. Lexi, the hot 21 year old server from the bar up the street was in there. I chatted her up and it was hard to focus with her in yoga pants and covered in sweat. She has a boyfriend but being young it can't be that serious. Could I pull it off? Maybe. Crazy to even think such a thing, but I want her. And she frightens the shit out of me.

This evening is injection time. I don't want Scarlett to see me so I'll do it while she is taking her bath. I think seeing her father injecting needles in his arm and belly would freak her out. It kind of freaks me out.

I weighed 181 yesterday at the gym. A little heavy for me. It's mostly in my gut. I think 172 is a good lean look for me. That may change now. I expect it to change. I'm only 5'7" so I do not carry a lot of weight on this frame.

After dinner my head clouded over and the pressure came back. I felt just a hint of depression. It's weird now. I'm not sad about anything. I can just feel the depression wash over me like a cloud. At least it is not as dark as it used to be. Not like in the bad Lyme days. Those were hell. This will be fine and gone tomorrow I expect. I am tired and feel like a good night's sleep is coming. Time to send Scarlett to the bath.

9:35 PM Once she was in the bath I got my stash of needles out of the cabinet and the HCG from the fridge and went to work. The damn testosterone was so thick in the insulin syringe that it took forever to get .5 mL in there. There is a tiny bubble that would not come out and I pictured it going in my blood vessel straight to my heart and me dying instantly in my kitchen. The nurse at the clinic said that won't happen but I bet it can. Shit. I swabbed my left shoulder good and popped it in and slowly depressed the plunger. My moustache tingled and got thicker I think as the oil began to circulate. The bubble stayed inside the syringe somehow and I dodged a bullet. This time.

I popped the HCG needle into my belly fat and barely felt a thing. Where will I put it when I'm all muscle and have .1% body fat? Maybe in my ass. There will always be some fat there. Or directly into my testicle. That sounds reasonable. I'll cross that bridge when I get there.

Everything is put away now and injection ceremony number 3 is complete. We will see what tomorrow brings.

10/20/17 Friday Day 9

I woke up at 2:33 AM wide awake. I lie there for 10 minutes and fell back to sleep. Not sure what that means if anything. I woke again at 3:34 cold, so I got up and turned the heat on. Then I slept soundly until 5:45. I wanted to get up and start my day, but I was sleeping so well that I went back to sleep. I had great morning wood at that point. Harder than any erection I have had in a good long while. I swear it was almost smiling at me.

Now it's 7:30 and I am up and my mind is clear. Barely any depression or anxiety this morning. I feel so relaxed I could climb back in bed and sleep some more. Maybe I will.

I am not sore at all from my workouts this week. My hips were a little stiff yesterday evening from the rowing I did. Probably used some muscles I don't normally use. But my chest is not sore like it normally is after a good workout, and my elbows don't hurt after doing pullups yesterday. I was really hoping this would help with inflammation and so far so good.

5:59 PM I have felt solid all day. I got good work done at home on the computer and knocked out a lot of my to do list. I went to the gym at lunch and did 2000M on the rowing machine again. This time I almost completed it in 9 minutes. I thought my biceps looked more vascular already, but I doubt there is much of an effect in only 9 days. This is not a steroid dose. I do feel better though. Placebo effect??

I called my nurse practitioner and asked her to reduce my depression meds by half. She agreed and I picked that up this afternoon. I stopped by Burke's Outlet while waiting on the script and there was a hot blonde with no wedding band on browsing around right where I walked in. I should have approached immediately, but I walked on by and it did not take long for the old excuses to show up for reasons I should leave her alone. "She probably has a boyfriend. I would just be bugging her. She is out of my league." One thing I really hope to rediscover from this journey is confidence. I chastised myself later for not just going up and saying hi. What's the worst that could happen?

Now I am back home and I am washing the new sheets and comforter I bought at Burkes. If I am going to have ladies over ever again, I want nice sheets.

My energy is stellar. Usually I am spent by now unless I have had an afternoon nap. But I could go for a jog if I wasn't going to have drinks with my friend Riley. No damn Jagermeister though. Just a couple of beers then call it a night. Hopefully.

11:34 PM Riley stood me up. So I went to mom and dad's and watched Blue Bloods and drank some of dad's whiskey. I knocked out 1000 words on the Lyme book before I went, along with a new blog post. I just feel real damn productive today. I hope this continues. It sucks having to dig deep for motivation. It would be nice to just wake up and get shit done every day. It seems like at one time I did. A long time ago. I am not sleepy but it's time for bed so I'm out. I look forward to another good day tomorrow.

10/21 Saturday Day 10
I slept great last night. I think I only got up to piss once. When I awoke after 8 hours I was refreshed and ready to go. I have to say having some of the brain fog lift is weird. I've been foggy and derealized for so long that returning to reality is kind of freaky. I have to be patient with myself during this time. When I got up I had no morning wood, but while I was lying in bed stretching and getting ready to rise I got wood. Weird.

Mom and dad picked me up and we went to the Mississippi State vs Kentucky game. I was a little uneasy on the ride down. I can't put my finger on what it was, just uneasy. Not really anxiety. Maybe adjusting to looking out the window and seeing fields that looked real and not like holograms. I shook it off and enjoyed the ride.

We ate at Mugshot's which was one of my favorite places when I lived there. I consider today a cheat day so I had a cheeseburger with fries and a couple of beers. It sat heavy in my belly. I felt goofy and spacey at the football game after that. Not bad, just not necessarily good. Emotionally flat might be the right way to describe it. I am wondering if the lower dose of antidepressant is already affecting my mood. Perhaps. I did catch myself ogling every decent looking girl there and wondering what she looked like under her clothes. At one point I had the thought that I need to get laid right now. That thought has not been present for a while.

My balls are drawn up today. Even with the HCG, they are definitely drawn up. Not sure what is up with that. I felt weird on the ride home. Maybe a little depression creeping back in. Nothing major, just enough to be noticed. I guess it's a marathon and not a sprint.

10/22 Sunday Day 11
I slept well last night, but woke up twice to pee. Neither was a long pee, but the urgency was there. I had no nocturnal wood and no morning wood. Disappointing. I was a bit brain foggy when I woke up but only slight depression or anxiety.

The sermon at church spoke to me about life being short and the days being precious. It confirms my decision to hopefully improve things with TRT. I can always go back to fighting fatigue, low libido, depression, and anxiety. I can sit in my recliner after work with no motivation, lingering in Lyme and watch life pass slowly by until I wake up and I am old and alone. Or not.

After church I packed for Ohio and drove north. I stopped at a restaurant to have lunch with the family. I wasn't hungry until I walked inside and smelled the food, and then I was suddenly ravenous. I filled my plate with vegetables and roast beef along with a separate salad plate. A good meal for a bodybuilder, even if I am only driving today. But I discovered they had pumpkin pie and I could not resist. Damn you pumpkin pie and your spicy deliciousness!

My mind began to clear up on the long drive north and I felt pretty good. Not a hint of anxiety or depression. Just comfortable being. Man this is enjoyable. I formed some vivid thoughts in my mind about the cute dental hygienist I'm interested in, but nothing really happened downstairs. I guess I was hoping for instant erections just by picturing someone naked, but it is not happening yet. Perhaps that is too much to ask.

I am currently listening to Robert Green's The Art of Seduction. It is an excellent book about human behavior and how people are seduced. It is not a pickup book but an examination of what motivates people and how to identify it and offer what is missing in their life. I can see the usefulness of this information if I can retain it.

The drive went by quickly and I stopped in Morehead, KY at a Hampton Inn for the night. The girl at the front desk was cute and flirted with me a little bit. I was friendly and flirted back and we talked about the Walking Dead for some reason. She suggested I watch Empire, whatever that is. In my mind I seduced her and she will let herself into my room when her shift is over. Any moment now. Or maybe I have to finish the Robert Green book first before I can pull that off. Maybe next stop.

I am completely comfortable and my mind and vision are clear. I have missed being able to just sit and type and just enjoy it. I appreciate the hard times in my life for forcing me to grow, but I appreciate the easy times much more now than I ever did before.

10/23 Monday Day 12
I stayed up until 1 AM reading and writing, then slept until 8AM. I am about to hit the road this morning and needed to get an early start but was sleeping so peacefully I gave myself an extra hour. I had semi-wood when I awoke. Better than nothing.

It is cold here in the hotel room and my boys are high and tight. I just completed my injections for the day. When I injected the HCG the needle did not go in easily and caused me to jump when it suddenly sunk past my tough skin. Damnit it hurt. Will TRT make me tougher? Surely I will scoff at pain in the near future.

I elected to put the T into my quad instead of my shoulder. Might as well share the love. I swabbed my left quad, or at least the area where a quad muscle should be. Damn my legs are skinny after Lyme. Time to get squatting again I guess. This one did not hurt and I watched in fascination as the thick liquid slowly penetrated my left thigh. I feel great and mighty now and I already put up my needles to be disposed of when I return home. I will now grunt at the ceiling, take a shower, and depart the hotel like a man.

1:11 PM The drive this morning was excellent. My vision is clear and sharp today, and I'd like to go to my optometrist and take the eye exam again to show him my eyes are fine. I had a checkup a couple of months ago and he said my vision was really deteriorating. I explained that I was recovering from Lyme and my vision changed day to day. He appeared not to believe me. But I can see like an effing hawk this morning so he can kiss my fat ass.

I continued listening to Robert Green on the drive up and was fascinated to learn of historical seducers and how they upended empires and governments. This is really an excellent book.

My mind is churning with thoughts of things I am going to knock out and get done. I am free and clear and determined. This is the way it should be. Not a trace of anxiety or depression. I am really liking this a lot.

Before I left, I ate scrambled eggs, cheerios, and a cup of yogurt at the hotel buffet. Not perfect but not terrible. I got a protein bar and Muscle Milk for lunch before I arrived at the plant. After work I'll go to the Marietta YMCA and have a nice leg workout. I have not worked them in a couple weeks so I cannot overdo it or there will be hell to pay. Just a solid and taxing workout and walk or bike for a bit afterwards. I look forward to it.

5:07 PM Earlier, sitting in the plant manager's office, I was keenly aware of the short skirt that the HR manager was wearing. Normally I would pay her no mind, but today I feel drawn to her. The sight of her legs excited me. I like this. Nothing was moving downstairs, but upstairs things seem to be active. Perhaps the early effects are mental and emotional and the physical comes later. We shall see.

And another weird thing happened. After the HR manager left I was suddenly hit with a wave of brain fog and a touch of depression. It was almost tangible. Not intense thank goodness, but definitely enough to get my attention. I wonder where this comes from. Lyme is a fickle bitch so it is difficult to determine if that is the culprit or the injection this morning. I'll keep an eye on this shit for sure.

10:10 PM I meditated for 10 minutes when I got back to the hotel and feel better now. Then I went to dinner with a colleague and was really talkative and confident during our conversation. Much more than usual. I could feel the flow. Maybe a little brain fog but I just went with it. I'm lying in bed now feeling pretty good. Ready for a complete night's sleep. I just feel like getting shit done. Only a couple weeks ago I was sleeping a lot in the afternoons and always tired. Maybe I'm not walking around with a permanent erection yet, but my energy and mood are definitely improved. TRT will be worth it for nothing else but those two, regardless if anything else improves. Good night.

10/24 Tuesday Day 13
I could not sleep last night. I was amped up when I got in bed, like I had drank a cup of coffee. Cortisol? Maybe. I just had energy. I listened to two sleep meditations from YouTube and finally drifted off to the second one, then woke again at 4:26am and that was it. I was wide awake. The good news is I did have a rock hard erection at that point. I took it out and wielded it like a lightsaber. Of course I did. I had been having a sexually frustrating dream about Pamela where we were in bed about to get it on but kept getting interrupted by various deterrents. I woke up just before I hit paydirt. Damnit. I always liked Pamela and that tight little body. If she is in my dreams then she will be in my arms soon enough. That's how it works, right?

At 6 I decided to hit the hotel fitness center and I ran a mile on the treadmill. I should say I jogged. My pace was over 10 minutes for one mile. Unacceptable. Still, I could have run further and felt solid overall. I got ready and had a solid breakfast of oatmeal and fruit with a small glass of milk and some eggs. I think that is a good start to my day.

The drive to work was very clear and purposeful. Really in a good place mentally. I turned off the radio and just talked to God most of the way. I don't do that enough. The colors seemed more vibrant in the fields along the interstate and the farms just radiated peace.

On a less positive note, my boys are riding very high and tight this morning. The actual testicle size appears normal, but my scrotum is pulled up tight like someone threw cold water on it. Weird. Maybe just adjusting to hormones? I did read online that HCG affects the scrotal volume or some shit like that. It seems to have different effects for different people. I even read that in pornos they give it to guys to make the nuts swell and look huge. Like those dudes need any help.

A weird thing that happened when I first got sick from Lyme, is my boys drew up like this. I attributed it to my body feeling under constant attack. I don't think that is the case now. I choose not to focus too much on it and just hope that they return to normal. I suppose it is not the end of the world if they don't hang low anymore, but I liked them the way they have always been.

1:54 PM It was a solid morning, but sometime before noon my head got a little fuzzy and a cloud just kind of washed across me. Not terrible. Nothing like the worst Lyme days. It just feels like I suddenly got knocked down a few notches on the joy scale. I actually smiled because it used to be so much worse. I am curious to see how TRT plays into this long term. I question its effect, if any, on my immune system and ability to keep the Lyme infection suppressed. My Lyme doctor had no issues with me starting it so I just have to trust the process. My boys have released a little and are now hanging lower, but not full like normal.

For lunch I had a salad with oil and vinegar dressing and a bowl of chili. Pretty good I think. I just finished a Quest protein bar for dessert. Those things are awesome. I wanted to workout last night but had to meet one of my bosses for dinner. I'll look for a hotel with a fitness center this evening.

Overall another solid day so far. Even now, I feel like doing something even with my mind a bit cloudy. So all is well.

11:44 PM I just made it to my hotel in Lexington, KY. I worked until 6:30 PM then hit the road and headed south. It was a good day of work. I did have a few mental hills to climb in the afternoon, but they really weren't bad. Just a bit of lingering depression that was more annoying than anything. I had 3 non-negative interactions with 3 different women. I had a text exchange with Kristi. She says she can't wait to see me, but I'm not too sure if she is really interested. I flirted over Facebook Messenger with Daphne, the young blonde I have had a few conversations with but never enough courage to push it anywhere. She is going to get back to me on something I posed to her. Maybe. And I called Jewel and talked. She can't wait for me to come see her, but sometimes I feel like I'm just a buddy to her. My boys are still drawn up this evening. I wonder if adjusting the HCG would help. Maybe change that to every other day. I'll give it a week and see. I was thinking some of it could be me sitting on my ass in a car for hours and hours on my trip this week. Maybe I'll fly to Chicago next week instead of driving to avoid a repeat. I suppose it's possible. I'd hate to get a bit insecure about my ball size with everything seemingly falling into place. Shit.

I snacked on protein bars on the drive down this evening and drank a Muscle Milk. I realized I am overeating a bit. I guess I really already knew that. It's time to track calories and cut some fat. My belly is just flabby right now. And stick to intermittent fasting. That has proved to be the most effective way for me to maintain a caloric deficit and steadily lose weight. I know subconsciously I am fearful of cutting back too much because when I got sick I was not eating enough. I was running a lot and stressing out and let my immune system get run down. But I should know that won't happen now. I learned from it and I listen to my body and I push when I can and rest as much as possible. Time for bed. I look forward to glorious morning wood and sweet dreams of Pamela. This time no damn interruptions.

10/25 Wednesday Day 14

No dreams of Pamela last night. I am awake after a solid 8 hours of mostly dreamless sleep. If Pamela was there I don't recall. Damnit.

I had decent morning wood. Not fully engorged, but it's hard and that is more than I was having just a few weeks ago. Mentally I am very clear with only a hint of anxiety or depression. Every morning should be so nice. I am impressed at the ability of testosterone to lift depression so quickly.

It was a beautiful day for a drive and I continued to listen to the Art of Seduction. Part of my journey to a new me is learning to communicate with women and charm the ones I am interested in. I have mostly been un-confident around women with the exception of a few years in high school and drunk college nights when I had some success. It's time to make a motherfucking change.

The drive was mostly uneventful with the exception of having to stop and pee every 45 minutes. I sure hope raising my estrogen levels helps with that eventually. Having to pee all the time sucks.

I stopped in Nashville at Smoothie King and got a Gladiator with peanut butter and bananas. I figure that is what a bodybuilder would drink. It tasted good and I felt my deltoids get bigger. Not.

Instead of going straight home I went to look at a 1966 Bronco. I have always wanted an old Bronco and this could be an opportunity. I can tell you my inner voices are giving me 101 reasons why making such a purchase is irresponsible. Why do those voices all sound like my dad? Before I even got there I saw an old Bronco sitting in a car dealership lot in some random small town in west Tennessee. I did a U-turn and went back to check it out. This rig was nice and solid. Not completely restored. A little rough inside. But a tough looking truck. The owner came out and told me it's his personal vehicle and not for sale. I was disappointed but figured just seeing an old Bronco while I am on my way to look at an old Bronco must be a sign.

I arrived around 3 PM and pulled into the lot that has the Bronco. There were several people checking it out which is not surprising. After checking it out myself, I am convinced of two things:

1. This is a good deal on the hottest selling collector vehicle in the country.
2. My limiting thoughts still fight me against doing something I really want to do.

After exchanging numbers with the owner, I left a little deflated that I am still unsure of myself. That I am still hesitant to jump into life and would rather watch from the sidelines. So fuck it. I decided to call the loan officer at my bank and get the payment info on a loan to purchase it. It comes out the same monthly payment as my car, which I am about to pay off. Another sign. I tell myself to sleep on it, but I already know I am doing this. The Bronco needs work, but nothing major. I can do most of it myself and have buddies who can do the rest. Time to jump in.

11:52 PM I am wide awake again. I had a killer leg workout this evening, then a healthy dinner of chicken salad sandwich and Kashi cereal with protein powder and almond milk. I got a haircut this afternoon and I swear my face looked fatter in the mirror. Maybe I am bloated? Not a good look for a soon to be lady killer. Tomorrow I will run and sweat. Hell, I have enough energy right now to run a 10k. I need to sleep though.

Tonight lying in bed I talked to my daughter in earnest for 10 minutes straight. Then it dawned on me that I had been talking to her for 10 minutes straight. Being caught up inside my own head for years has kept my conversations to a minimum. Guess I better get used to having something to say.

This afternoon as I was getting ready to head to the gym, I felt my mood begin to shift and I caught it. I stopped mid stride and just observed it. By being aware of it, it dissipated. Weird. The mind is a funny ass thing.

One positive note is after riding high most of the day I noticed my boys were hanging low when I was getting ready for bed. Maybe it was just riding in the car for hours and they needed some blood flow. I have yo-yo balls now. Nice.

10/26 Thursday Day 15

I was able to go to sleep last night just after midnight, then I slept like a rock for 8 hours. I slept through the alarm and caused Scarlett to be late for school. But man it was good sleep. And when I awoke I was instantly full of energy and ready to tackle the day. That feeling has been gone since probably high school. Makes me realize how shitty my sleep has been over the years. I'll get a handle on the night time energy. Could be related to the late evening leg workout. Maybe try and hit it earlier in the day. We'll see.

My morning wood was delayed again. It was not there when I first woke up, but when I walked into the closet to throw on some jeans and take my daughter to school, morning wood suddenly appeared like magic. I'll take it. So what that tells me is I'll need to get out of bed first to have morning sex. The sacrifices one makes...

My boys are back up tight this morning but it is cold outside and drafty inside so that is not helping. I'm thinking of moving the HCG to 3 X week and not on my testosterone injection days. Worth a try. Mentally I feel so good this morning I could cry. Just nothing but love for the world. So many days spent suffering through Lyme these past couple of years. And decades of anxiety and mental fog before I even got sick. This is so much better, and I am just getting started!

9:11 PM Well, I have concluded that I might possibly be a dumbass. I did my injection tonight while Scarlett was back in her room. I injected the .5 mL just like I have been. The liquid was thick and took forever to load and to plunge into my shoulder. I glanced at the box the testosterone came in and noticed is said .5 mg, or .25 mL Shit! I've been giving myself a double dose! No telling what my damn testosterone is right now. Estrogen too!

No wonder I have so much energy and went from half dead to crushing it in the gym. I even tried to have an anxiety attack but I'm too mentally calm and focused to have one apparently. All I could do was laugh at myself. I'll be sure and hit the gym hard tomorrow and take advantage of this blast before I come back down. The shit I get myself into.

10/27 Friday Day 16

I slept great last night. I drifted off a little after 10 and woke up at 5:45 AM ready to wrestle bears. I got up and meditated and wrote some and planned my day. I made Scarlett breakfast and packed her lunch and we got ready on time. The whole morning I felt great, but I did get a little bit of brain fog mid-morning. High estrogen? Stress from double dosing? Probably both. I still feel great though so I will just ride this out and learn from it.

I had zero morning wood so I tried to work up an erection in the shower. It took some doing but I finally got one that was not my best work. I did not finish. I just wanted to see what I could do. Maybe tomorrow will be better. Patience is the key word here.

I did go to the gym around noon and hit my chest hard. And of course the weight I've been using seemed easy and I was able to go up quite a bit. It felt good and I got something I had forgotten about in the gym: a real pump. My pecs were tight in my shirt and I could feel the blood pumping. It's been a few years since I felt that. It felt good. I had to cut it a bit short to go to an event at the church, but I could have worked out all afternoon. I also weighed in and I have gained 3 lbs. I'm sure it is water weight. I do feel bloated and my pants were tight this morning. I have not eaten enough to gain 3 lbs of fat or muscle, so it's mostly water. Perhaps when I get on a normal dose of testosterone my hormones will settle down and I can release some water.

I also noticed that my left ear is not ringing so loud. It's still there, but not as noticeable. I'm down to the lowest dose of the antidepressant and my mood is 95% positive. I think those meds cause some tinnitus in some people. Man I hate that damn ringing.

Tonight I have people coming over to hang out at my house and I am excited. I've been living here for 3 years and can count on one hand the times I have invited people over for a social. I really look forward to entertaining guests and having conversation. Shit, did I just write that? Who is this guy? I like him.

10/28 Saturday Day 16

I woke up with great morning wood today! I mean Mr. Wiggly was like a flagpole. It felt so awesome! I just lie there in bed admiring it. Hell, I thought about snapping a selfie. I had truly forgotten what it is like to awake with great morning wood. And I had a few beers last night which seemed to have no negative effect.

I mustered up the courage and bought the damn Bronco. I have wanted one for so long. I decided to quit being a wuss and just do it. Yes, there are plenty of reasons why buying a 50 year old vehicle makes no sense. I can hear the thoughts in the back of my mind. Those limiting thoughts that try and keep us where we are. But I am determined to break through those. TRT is a part of that journey as I learn to live with no anxiety and the confidence of renewed masculinity. And this alpha male wants a 1966 Bronco.

Last night I found myself so confident I thought I could actually turn a lesbian straight. There was a cute blonde one here hanging out at my gathering and she and I had fun talking. I'm sure she has an effect on all men, but she sucked me in pretty quick. The thing is, I felt like I really built rapport. Like if it was just me and her I might could have made something happen. I'm probably dreaming but at least my thought pattern is shifting in the right direction. Better than thinking she would never have me.

Yesterday evening at the market I was very flirty with the two blonde checkout girls. There were both around 20 I'd say, and I'm 42 but I know one of them responded. The other one not so much. I'll take 50%. Hell I almost invited her to my gathering, but I instead let it slip that I was cooking dinner for people to make it sound like I am in demand. Perhaps I set the stage for a later encounter. This pickup and seduction stuff is so counterintuitive. Time to go get the Bronco.

11:11 PM This was a nice day. This afternoon I took a nap and as I lie there drifting off, it suddenly occurred to me that I had a raging erection! What the hell? This is like teenage shit. I even looked under the covers to admire my stiff one. It was glorious. It is time to share this gift with the world.

Usually I skip a day between workouts, but I have been feeling strong so I went ahead and did my back and biceps routine ahead of schedule. Again I got a hell of a pump. My biceps and lats were bulging. My lats have not bulged since college. Also, I'm still up 3 lbs. But I look more muscular now. I'm glad I caught the double dose of T or I would have some explaining to do pretty quickly as I morphed into a little Hercules. I have been a little foggy here and there today. Maybe high estrogen? I still felt great though. Zero anxiety. It's like it does not exist in my mind or body any more. No depression either. A few times I kind of zoned out emotionally, but that is as likely Lyme related as anything. This is all so much better than what I have faced daily for the past couple of years.

The real challenge right now is adjusting to feeling good and positive vs fighting for dear life or wanting to die at certain points. It's a hell of a swing. Just take it a day at a time. Shit's about to get real fun.

10/29 Sunday Day 17
I woke up after 8 hours of solid sleep. I feel rested when I wake up now. For 30 years or so I have woken up still tired no matter how much sleep I got. This is a welcome change after only a few weeks.

I had decent morning wood today. Not great but decent. After yesterday's midday surprise I was expecting to wake up and drive nails, but I'll settle for decent wood. I went to church and found I was a bit foggy during the sermon. Just enough to notice. But I was in a good place emotionally and felt connected to everyone in the sanctuary. I felt love. It was nice.

After that, Scarlett and I came home and had lunch then I got sleepy for some reason. I took about an hour nap while she went with my mother shopping. I woke up feeling great again. I suppose I could have skipped the nap, but I had an afternoon to myself so why not? I considered the gym but after two hard days in a row I wisely decided to rest. I just got over years of battling Lyme disease after all.

I drive to Chicago tomorrow for the week. I look forward to continuing listening to the Art of Seduction. Plus I have meetings with 3 of the hottest women I have ever encountered when I get there. 2 blondes just out of college and 1 brunette around 30 with a tight ass. I would have actually dreaded meeting with them before due to the intimidation factor, but now I look forward to dazzling them with my bullshit. What a difference a few weeks makes. If I hook up with one of them I'll be so high no one could bring me down. I'll be unstoppable.

This is a chance to gain experience travelling with my injection kit. I'm driving so it's not so difficult, but still I have to keep the HCG shot on ice until I get there and the testosterone shot is preloaded and must be cared for.

I went ahead and took my HCG today instead of in the morning. I am going to start injecting it the day before my test instead of all on the same day. I read on Excelmale.com that others are doing this and having success, so I'll give it a try. Perhaps it will keep my boys hanging more consistent.

10/30 Monday Day 18
I felt weird last night before I fell asleep. A little anxious, but it was a different kind of anxiety. Just an uneasiness that I could not quite sort out. I fell asleep okay, but awoke in the middle of the night with a feeling of dread. It really sucked. I went back to sleep and slept soundly until 6 AM, then got up and had some coffee and began writing. I felt pretty okay at that point. No morning wood though and my boys were drawn up tight. Not a good feeling.

After my coffee a slight fog settled over my awareness. It was different than the usual brain fog. It was like everything was in kind of slow motion. Hard to describe, but not normal. I let it go and decided to be okay with it.

I did my testosterone injection before I left. I decided to do it in my left quad for whatever reason. I bled like a damn stuck pig. I must have hit a capillary or something. It quit bleeding pretty quickly though so I guess I'll survive.

10:43 PM It was a tough drive to Chicago. I did not leave until around 11 AM because I had some work to do at the house. I felt so uneasy about leaving. It just felt all wrong. In the past I would have said the feelings were leading up to a big old panic attack. But it never came. I just felt wired to the gills and not like myself. I had a thought that it was kind of like taking a shot of cocaine without the bliss. It dissipated after a couple of hours and the drive was nice for a short period. Fields of cows and crops and little farms. I found myself saying the words "I am happy". Weird thing to say I suppose, but it could be worse.

But then my stomach began to cramp up. Really bad. My belly blew up so big that my chest hurt and my lungs were tight. My bladder had so much pressure that I nearly pissed myself. Something caused a hell of a reaction in my stomach. All I had on the road were protein bars, Muscle Milk, and protein cookies. Not sure what did it. Too much processed food, perhaps. Or the shredded wheat biscuits I ate the night before catching up with me. But it made for a miserable drive. Pain for hours in my chest, stomach, and gut. I stopped to shit once and it helped, but not enough. I had to piss every 20 minutes due to the terrible pressure on my bladder, so it took forever to get here.

I feel better now. My head is a little clearer and my belly has deflated. I look forward to a good night's sleep. Jewel and Kristi have both been texting me, and I like having women seem interested in me again. Maybe I'll have the courage to get inside one or the other of them soon.

10/31 Tuesday Day 19
I slept hard last night. I put on a sleep meditation and heard maybe the first two minutes and I was out. I got up once to pee then right back to sleep. My alarm went off at 6 AM but I was not motivated to get up and kick ass. Just sleeping too well.

I lie there and evaluated my mood and it was a bit low. Not depressed but low. I let it be for a while and did some deep breathing and visualization then felt better. I got up and noticed I looked leaner and more muscular in the hotel mirror. I guess skipping dinner last night due to the bloating allowed my puffiness to subside.

I had morning wood when I awoke, but it was not too hard and kind of skinny. Not full at all. Not what I wanted, but better than a wet noodle I suppose. My boys were drawn up pretty high. It's weird, the actual ball size seems pretty normal they are just being pulled up high by the cords that attach them. A hell of a design God had there.

Once I got up and got my shower, my mood lifted and I was ready to get to work and get shit done. I am in the office in Chicago feeling froggy and ready to hop.

It's Halloween night and I am staying in downtown Chicago. If a man can't get laid in that environment, then perhaps he just cannot get laid. I plan on going out tonight and definitely talking to the ladies. We'll see what happens.

11:38 AM I just had a revelation. For the past couple weeks I have gotten back into intermittent fasting, which I know helps me to lose weight quickly. I also recall that when I used to do this I would feel cold and my balls would draw up, precisely as they are doing now. Maybe it is not the testosterone or HCG but the lack of food in the morning and the cortisol spike I probably get when I drink coffee on an empty stomach. Tomorrow I will eat a healthy breakfast and have half a cup of coffee. I am hopeful that my boys emerge from their hidey hole once they see it is safe to come out and my body is no longer in fight or flight.

10 PM I had a nice workout this evening. The hotel gym had a decent setup. I did leg presses and leg curls since I only had 30 minutes. My legs felt strong, but my right knee is acting up. Have to watch that. My mood is solid. Zero anxiety and no depression even though I forgot to take my antidepressant today. I am so ready to be done with those. I feel better not

having taken it, but I took it just now because I am not ready to quit cold turkey. Maybe in the next 30 days or so.

At dinner tonight I was spot on with conversation. At one point I even became aware of the fact that my normal filter telling me to stay guarded and quiet was not there. I was conversational, flirty with my coworker Kate, alpha talking with my former boss Richard, and overall I enjoyed the company. In the past I would have been content to drink and eat alone while reading or writing. I like being sociable. And the waitress, while a hefty gal, was very into me. She went out of her way to help me figure out where the best Halloween parties were. Very chatty. Hefty gals need love too!

11/1 Wednesday Day 20
I woke up with an erection so hard I could chop wood with it. It was a thing of beauty. And my boys were hanging lower and pretty full. There appears to be no rhyme or reason to this, although I know from a physiological perspective there has to be. Hopefully I can pinpoint it.

I slept like a rock again. Dreamless sleep for about 6.5 hours. When I awoke I was rested but not wide awake nor ready to tackle the day. I hit the snooze and meditated until the timer went off. Then I got up feeling pretty froggy.

I ate a solid breakfast at the hotel cafe. Oatmeal, scrambled eggs, plain Greek yogurt, and some pineapple. And a small cup of coffee. Should last me until lunch time.

The 3 attractive consultants I am meeting with today arrive sometime after lunch. I am curious to see how my confidence is around them or if I shrink away and get intimidated. Normally I would be intimidated and have to get drunk in order to feel comfortable around such company, but today I want to just relax and let them know me and hear what I have to say. I hope it goes well.

6:11 PM Our afternoon meetings went just fine. All of the beautiful women were so happy to see me and we enjoyed joking and being in each other's company. It was so different than most of my experiences with beautiful women. We got some solid work done and then parted ways.

I just did my HCG injection in my hotel room. It's been in the mini fridge since I got here and it's nice and cold. I noticed a big ass bubble headed towards my belly fat just as I finished the plunge. Shit. If it went into my fat what will happen? Got to figure out how to get these bubbles out. My boys are hanging better already just from eating breakfast this morning. I'm about to head to the gym then a night on the town. Should be fun.

11:11 PM It was a great night. I got a little drunk without meaning to, but not bad. Kate, Richard, and I had dinner at a fancy seafood place, then I insisted we go to the House of Blues. In the past I would have been the first one to want to go back to the hotel and get away from crowds and social settings, but tonight I just felt on. I wanted to be out and around people. I can't even believe I'm writing this. Even in college I had some social anxiety and did not always enjoy going out. This is so different, and in such a short amount of time. I cannot tell much difference in my body composition yet, but my mood has changed within a few weeks. What will happen in a few months?

My workout was nice tonight before we left. I felt strong and focused, and wanted to lift more but my shoulders hurt. Just a bit of impingement. I need to do more stabilizing exercises.

11/2 Thursday Day 21
I woke up at 5:30 AM with a damn hangover. I stayed in bed until 6:30 and still had a hangover when I got up. But I was able to shake it off pretty quickly and get going. Once I got out of bed I was pretty okay. By the time I got a shower I was ready to roll. I really should pay a higher price for my night out, but damn I've got good energy already. Oh well. Hangovers hurt less with high testosterone. Who knew?

I also woke up with a rock hard erection and a decent hang to my balls. Not a bad start. I can't wait to get to work and see the consultant girls. They are all so cute. Maybe they'll show me their boobs. It could happen.

11:46 PM Not a bad day at all. I was extremely busy and very focused and full of energy. My confidence was sky high, and I enjoyed conversing and flirting with the consultant girls. Shit, I would have been extremely intimidated by them in the past, thinking of all the reasons they would never have me. Today I was just thinking that I want to mount one of them. Very primal. I swear one of them was shaking her ass at me and poking her breasts out at me. Damn they all looked good.

Even with my lack of sleep and slight hangover, I was never really tired today. I ate a good breakfast, then a healthy lunch at Whole Foods. I just felt good. No brain fog. No depression. I am loving this. How good can it get? Kristi texted me and we made a date for Monday. After two years of hell a lot is just falling into place. About time.

11/3 Friday Day 22
I got up late in Paducah, KY and drove home barely in time to see Scarlett in her play. Her mother had failed to bring her choir uniform to school and Scarlett was so embarrassed she was the only one in plain clothes. I was pissed.

Normally I would have let it go and just tried to get along for the sake of not fighting with my ex, but I felt like I had to speak my mind on this one. Her mother fucked up and I wanted justice. So I told her mother how I felt and how much it hurt her daughter.

At first she tried to blame everyone under the sun. That woman absolutely hates being accountable for her actions. But I made my thoughts known clearly and rationally and did not lose my cool. She eventually apologized and admitted she was having a bad day. How about that? Is this what winning looks like?

Several of us went out to a bar tonight and drank beer until midnight. There was a 19 year old waitress there who is so damn smoking hot it is difficult to look at her without getting blinded.

In the past I would have avoided eye contact and kept my distance for fear of being shamed by her beauty, but this time I asked someone for her name and called out to her to get me a beer please. She smiled at me so big my dick did a cartwheel right there. When she brought the beer I made a wisecrack about the ugly ass Ole Miss cap she had on and instead of firing back she immediately began making excuses and offered to wear a Mississippi State hat if I would bring her one. I'll be damned. She is one of the hottest girls I have ever seen in person but around me she was the one less confident. What kind of Jedi mind trickery is this?

As I continue to overcome depression, anxiety, physical illness, and a life of average confidence, I'll ponder the odds of successfully seducing a 19 year old hottie at 42 years of age. That would be the most epic sex story of my life to date, but perhaps in the end it will be one of many.

11/4 Saturday Day 23
I felt like shit this morning. Drank way too many beers last night, even though it was like 7 total. I'm just not a big drinker anymore thank goodness. Still, I got 6 solid hours of sleep and woke up with pretty good energy. Not long ago someone would have to drag me out of bed.

I went to a football game with mom and dad. On the drive down I felt hungover and I realized something pretty profound. For all of my adult life a hangover equaled instant anxiety. But as we rode back roads through small towns on our way to Starkville, there was not an ounce of anxiety in my body. It was almost uncomfortable. Anxiety was such a huge part of me for so long, it's like losing a piece of myself and it takes some adjustment to get used to it being gone. But I can definitely get used to this.

At the ballgame I noticed every young hot girl within a 100 yard radius. Like I could catch their scent or something. I think a couple of them even gave me a good look. Interesting after only a few weeks. Perhaps it was wishful thinking. There were a few girls that were so hot and wearing such tight fitting clothes that I felt like I had to have them right then and there. A very urgent need that I have not felt in years. Have to keep an eye on that and determine how to channel it into something productive.

The game was fun and my buddy gave me a little Scotch to take the edge off. I felt better after that, so I drank a couple of beers on the ride home. Then I got home and started wondering if I was becoming an alcoholic and it freaked me out a little. So I took a nap.

I awoke in a fog and did not feel good at all. My breathing felt labored and I just felt sluggish. I worried that I had weakened my body and Lyme was coming back. Not a good feeling. I commit to drinking much less and exercising more and eating healthy. I refuse to go back to being sick.

11/5 Sunday Day 24
I woke up feeling much better. Still a bit foggy, but overall better. My boys were hanging nice and low but no morning wood. Oh well.

I ate a breakfast of oatmeal and whey powder, then had a big lunch of roast beef and fresh vegetables at my mother's. I felt so bloated and fat I was miserable. Could barely button my pants. Damnit it's time to lose some belly fat.

Scarlett got back from her weekend with her mom and we watched Hallmark Christmas movies. It was nice being able to watch them and enjoy them again. Last Christmas I was so sick I barely remember anything about the holiday season.

I noticed my sport coat at church was tight through the shoulders. Am I already putting on muscle? I weighed 185 the other day which is heavy for me. 175 is a much better look and feel, but perhaps that will change as I add muscle to my frame. I really want to do complete a good leg workout. I will make it happen this week hopefully.

11/6 Monday Day 25
I feel emotionally flat this morning. I had a wet dream last night which was interesting, and awoke with decent morning wood. I'm not really horny though. Hard to say if this is Lyme or hormones. Maybe both. I was initially told it would take maybe 10 years to fully recover from Lyme. But I made progress at a good rate compared to many of my doctor's patients,

and I just refused to accept that 10 years of my life would be spent in agony. I would never last that long. I would end it. But I'm better and getting better every day. The trick now is knowing what symptoms are still fucking with me and being able to not only accept it but distinguish it from any irregularities from hormonal imbalances. So fucking complicated is my life. But I am thankful to still have it.

The drive to kickass and get shit done that had been building is now diminished quite a bit. Just a blah feeling that I need to shake. Perhaps it is related to the drinking. I look forward to drying out this week and getting back to a clear mind.

I'm eating Kashi cereal with whey powder and almond milk with my coffee this morning. I think that is pretty healthy. I hope to get to the gym later since I did not go yesterday. It is leg day, but my right knee is feeling a bit weak. Have to watch that.

My boys are hanging decent this morning. They have been since I started eating breakfast again. I wonder what that response is? Maybe cortisol related. Last night they were hanging really low, fuller than they have been in months. These damn balls of mine.

IS THIS GOING ANYWHERE?

11/7 Tuesday Day 26

I slept like a damn rock last night. Out at about 10:30 PM, and up at 5:45 AM ready to wrestle bears. Decent morning wood. I did not have to get up and pee once during the night. When is the last time that happened?

I feel a bit more motivated today. Perhaps yesterday was just an off day. I saw a post by some dude on the Facebook TRT Page of how he looked after 3.5 years. He looked like a damn hulk. He hinted that he also blasted some during this time, and said he felt better now than he did when he was 20. The guy is my age.

The thought of blasting is an interesting concept. I have enough testosterone to do that for 6-8 weeks probably. Admittedly I don't have the knowledge today, but it is available should I choose to do so. If I did that I'm pretty sure people would know I'm on something. Maybe I'll consider it down the road after the full results of TRT are evident.

My boys continue to hang low. I am testing this fasting hypothesis again. Today I will fast until noon. I was making a bit of progress leaning out until I began eating breakfast again. After only a few days my pants got tighter and I felt fatter. Damn breakfast. I know intermittent fasting is an excellent tool for not just leaning out but for all kinds of other health benefits, but does it truly cause balls to draw up? This time I am limiting the coffee on an empty stomach to half a cup or less and see if that helps.

Another observation I have is that my eyebrows, which had already thinned after Lyme disease, appear to be even thinner these past few weeks. My thyroid numbers were great at last check, but it's something to continue to monitor going forward. I'll ask the Lyme doc run more labs tomorrow when I go for my checkup.

I did acupuncture yesterday for the ringing in my ears and the neck and shoulder stiffness. It was pretty cool and my neck and shoulders definitely hurt less when I left. Not sure about any change in the ringing. The old Chinese doctor said it would take a while on the ringing but it would work. I hope so. That ringing pisses me off. But insurance doesn't cover it and that shit ain't cheap. It would be worth it to cure the ringing though.

I have a date with Kristi tonight, but I am not as excited as I should be. I suddenly feel out of her league. Now that's a damn 180 from a few years ago. I have been doing some reading on pickup and seduction and it has me feeling like Don Juan. We'll see if she immediately takes her panties off and hands them to me when we meet.

8:33 PM Kristi cancelled our date. Said her son got sick. Maybe, but who knows. I sent her a reply text stating that I understood and we would re-schedule for another time, but she did not respond. Weird girl. I'm not feeling too froggy anyway.

The motivation I thought I found this morning has waned over the course of the day. I feel kind of blah. I admittedly felt better when I was mistak-enly taking double the dose of Test. Perhaps I feel better at higher levels. I'll discuss that with the clinic when I go back. My desire to write or pick up around the house or go to the gym or meet women is pretty low right now. In fact, I could probably just go on to bed and sleep. I felt pretty unstoppable those first couple of weeks. Maybe tomorrow will be better.

Also, I have made a deal with myself that there is no fap until I have sex with a woman. So I am hoping that motivates me to get off my ass and find a girl. I missed a real chance this morning at the acupuncturist's office. A damn cute girl was flirting with me and I did not even pick up on it until I was called back to the waiting room. I was too caught up in my own head wishing I could meet a cute girl like that, and hell there she was talking to me about random shit and smiling and being overly friendly. Shit, some-times I wonder how I ever got laid.

11/7 Tuesday Day 27
I feel emotionally flat again this morning. Very foggy. No morning wood.

I only slept about 5.5 hours as I had to wake up early and drive 2.5 hours to see my Lyme doctor. He said I had made an amazing recovery and to stay on path. To keep my immune system strong keep taking the herbal tinctures that treat Lyme. I swear this shit doesn't feel real sometimes. How in the hell can there be a disease that has no real cure and people are left to rely on herbal shit when their antibiotic cocktails don't completely eliminate the infection? The fuckers at the CDC and IDSA should be prosecuted for crimes against humanity. I am one of the lucky ones.

I felt foggy and distant on the drive back. Still no anxiety, but maybe a bit of depression creeping in. Definitely a diminished drive and no feeling of libido. Although I admit it is hard to judge libido in the absence of a woman. Still, my package seemed pretty lifeless and I had no morning wood and no arousal throughout the morning.

7:33 PM After coming home and sitting on the couch and feeling depression sweep over me, I pulled my shit together and went to the gym and did a great full body workout. I immediately felt better. I worked up a good sweat and my legs were shaky afterward. I had a hell of a pump, something I am still getting used to. I can recall working out a few years ago and really pushing myself in the gym and no pump. It was so defeating.

I did my HCG injection before I went. I did double the dose since I will miss the next one. I am leaving tomorrow to go hunting with dad for a week and although I could take a loaded syringe and keep it in the fridge at camp, I am not ready to divulge to family that I am on TRT. Perhaps after I become a little Hercules with a full beard I will have no choice, but for now it will be between me and the clinic. The injection hurt for some reason. I must have found a tough spot in my belly fat.

There were three young hotties at the gym and I flirted a bit with two of them. I did not know the 3rd. And it just dawned on me that the two I flirted with have boyfriends. So why the hell didn't I talk to the other one? I have much to learn.

Now that I am home and all pumped up, I feel motivated and my emotions are relaxed and content. I have been packing for our deer hunting trip and feeling mentally clear and ready to roll.

Exercise is important to wellbeing. Who knew?

11/9/17 Thursday Day 28
Four weeks on TRT. The biggest improvement to date is my mood. Although I have been a little flat these past few days, overall my mood is much better. No wood this AM.

I do feel a bit stronger in the gym, but there could be some placebo there. My workouts had become so lifeless as I struggled through Lyme with low T. Now I know there is T running in my veins and I feel purpose again when moving the weight.

I do hope to get some confidence with women back. I feel so useless around them now. It's all wishful thinking at this point. Even before Lyme I was pretty ineffective. I was just ready to settle for someone who might spend some time with me.

I woke up at 5:50 AM this morning before my alarm, feeling wide awake and ready to get shit done. My mind was clear and I was in a good mood. No body aches and no sore throat, so Lyme is at bay. The only thing missing was a good morning woody. Where has that gone? Perhaps I'll do better on a higher dose since I started off with great results at 200 mg/week. I guess we'll find out in a couple of weeks when I do my first blood draw.

Looking down at my arm I can see the beginning of a bicep. I had such muscular arms in my 20's. Women used to compliment them and want to feel them. Then at some point they thinned out and got soft, no matter how many curls I did. It will be nice to feel out a shirt again.

Jewel texted me a pic of her panties, and gave me her bra and panty size in case I wanted to buy her some erotic clothing. Shit, I've got to get down to the coast and see that woman. That is guaranteed hot sex, assuming I can perform. Could I pull it off? I'm just not sure. The last time we were together I lasted about 5 minutes and could not get it up for a second act. It was so damn disappointing because she looked so damn good and was ready to fuck all night. Next time will be better I hope.

Scarlett is up so time to get ready for work and school. Time to go to work.

11/10/17 Friday Day 29
I woke up with a major erection this morning. I am in Columbia, MO on my way to deer hunt in Cainesville, and we stopped over at an Airbnb rental.

I did my injection last night. No HCG. I did not want the hassle of trying to keep it refrigerated on this hunting trip, so we'll see how I do without it.

Mentally I feel pretty good this morning. We stayed up too late shooting the shit and drinking whiskey, but it doesn't seem to affect me as much right now.

We ate dinner at a local pub down the street, and I was very flirty with the owner's daughter who served us. She was all smiles and seemed to enjoy me carrying on with her. My confidence is growing but has miles to go. The whole situation was dream like. This will take some adjustment for sure.

11/11/17 Saturday Day 30
We are at our hunting lodge in Cainesville. I use the term lodge loosely. We are actually staying in the guide's parents' basement. It's pretty cramped but there appear to be lots of big deer in the area.

There is a group of men from Michigan hunting here also. I enjoyed meeting them last night and comparing stories and backgrounds. In the past my social anxiety would have kept me from participating as much, but I was yucking it up with the best of them. I would have entered a pissing contest had I been challenged.

I slept well and woke up at 4 AM ready to hunt. I can recall for decades my dad having to drag me out of the bunk to go hunting. Last night I closed my eyes, slept for the allotted time, and woke up ready to go. And with a damn fine boner I might add. That is several days in a row now. I hope this continues and becomes the new norm.

11/12/17 Sunday Day 31
Another day of hunting. I missed a big buck this morning. Not sure what happened.

Last night we watched MSU vs Alabama and MSU almost pulled off the upset. They would have had the refs not protected Alabama down the stretch, but no one was surprised to see that happen. Even the Michigan boys who watched it with us said it was very lopsided by the refs. Oh well.

I felt very aggressive during the game. Something about getting excited and drinking whiskey with men and cussing and yelling. My dad's buddy Lawrence got drunk and was being aggravating and I found myself wanting to shove him or slap him. It was weird. I even raised my voice to him in a pissed off manner once which I have never done. He seemed to get the message and left me alone.

I went to bed angry at the loss and woke up sleepy at 5 AM. With a rock hard erection. I am on a roll. It would be just lovely to share these with a woman. Perhaps soon.

My boys are also hanging quite low even without the HCG. I am eating a good breakfast each morning and that seems to do the trick. What the hell is the correlation with breakfast and scrotum size? I like fasting because I can lean out quickly, but I like my balls too. This is madness.

11/13/17 Monday Day 32
Another day of hunting. It was cold and foggy this morning and I only saw 3 does. Bucks aren't moving for shit. Everyone is at camp right now napping but I have good energy. I just did my T injection and my shoulder bled quite a bit. Weird.

I noticed some lifting of brain fog in the past couple of days. It seems to go in steps instead of gradually. Like I stay at one level of fog and then I feel something weird going on inside my head and another layer dissipates. I am very close to zero fog which would be nice. Derealization is quickly dissipating. I had almost forgotten what the world really looks like. Although this is nice it is also kind of scary. Too much reality is sometimes not a good thing.

I reduced my antidepressant dose to every other day. I am ready to get off that shit. I feel so much better emotionally now I am positive I will be okay without the meds.

I did feel some anxiety yesterday evening in the deer stand. Just a bit to remind me what it's like. It quickly passed. Then I got it again walking into Walmart after dinner. But it passed in only a few seconds. It's like the anxiety is trying to tell me something, but since I am not afraid of it then it does not stick around.

This morning I had another great erection. I am ready to see Jewel. She called me last night and I found myself fantasizing about her when I went to bed and again this morning in the deer stand. This damn no fap November is for the fucking birds, but I remain strong. I may blow a gasket, but I am steadfast in my commitment. I just need some damn pussy. Did I just type that??

No anxiety at all today. And no depression at all either. Just a good old feeling of being okay and ready to get shit done when this hunting trip is over. And maybe ready to call on women again. Maybe.

11/14 Tuesday Day 33
I did my injection last night before bed. No HCG, just the T. My boys are drawn up pretty good today, and I have been eating plenty for breakfast. Does it happen that fast with no HCG?

My morning wood was more like morning flexible pipe today. Not hard but not flaccid. My mind has been clear though and my mood very good.

When all the guys are around camp I find myself getting in on the conversations instead of hanging around the edges just listening. Damn I spent a lot of years not even knowing I had social anxiety. I was always participating in my head. It would surprise me sometimes for people to describe me as quiet when I felt like I was always talking. Just talking inside my head.

So my results so far are excellent for mood and confidence. I'm eating quite a bit on this hunt but not sure I have gained any more weight. Maybe that tapers off after the first few weeks. I'll weigh in at the gym when I get back. I feel fuller in the back and shoulders.

Also, I have not shaved in 5 days. I have tried in vain over the years to grow a beard but never could get it to come in on my cheeks. A goatee is no problem, and even then my lower jaw and neck grow okay, but not on the cheeks. I hope that will change eventually, but what I see so far are the same hairless patches on my cheeks. I will say that the hair on my neck and lower jaw is much darker and coarser then it was previously. Perhaps a bit thicker as well. But my cheeks remain defiant. Damnit.

Lawrence made a comment that he woke up to pee last night and I was snoring loud as a bear. Is this getting worse? I'll use one of those snore apps to get an idea of this. Maybe I need a sleeping mouthpiece or something. Hopefully I am not ready for a CPAP yet.

11/15 Wednesday Day 34

No erection at all today. Where did it go? And my balls are up very high. The actual ball size is still pretty much full - they are just being pulled up tight like I've been in a cold bath. I picture a little gremlin inside pulling on my ball strings and having a big old time at my expense. Fucking gremlins.

I have spent hours in deer stands these past several days, and passed a lot of that time by fantasizing about women. I found I could easily get an erection any time I wanted by just visualizing the scene. That has not always been the case these past few years. But today I did not feel in the mood. That's a weird thing to say. I was just bored sitting in a tree watching squirrels, and I had no desire to picture naked women in my mind. Not sure if that means anything but it's definitely a change.

My overall mood is still solid though. No depression or anxiety. In a positive place with a good outlook on the future. I just feel like getting shit done and taking care of business. I'm just motivated without having to drag my ass along. I like that feeling.

11/16 Thursday Day 35
None of us killed a deer. That stinks. We paid roughly $9k between the 3 of us for this hunt and are going back empty handed. We did find a better place to hunt just down the road that we will probably come to next year, but this year was a letdown.

Still, I felt a shit ton better than I did a year ago in Kansas hunting. I was so damn sick and in so much pain then from Lyme that I should have been home in bed. And I was severely depressed and had no business sitting alone for hours with a loaded rifle in my hand. But I survived. In pain. Only ibuprofen and Jack Daniels got me through that damn trip. This year I could at least enjoy sitting in the woods and shooting the shit around camp.

No morning wood today. Will it come back? I think my labs are due to be drawn next week. Will my estradiol be high? I doubt it. It's always been low along with low free T. It should finally be creeping up into range. I will recheck my thyroid as well to see if the T is affecting it.

So no morning wood and no feelings of horniness, but my damn balls are hanging nicely today. WTF?? I haven't had HCG in over a week and they decide to suddenly hang down in total defiance? Damn ball gremlin at it again.

I did the driving most of the way back and my head was clear. No anxiety or depression. My vision was kind of blurry though. It was often blurry during my sickest Lyme days but mostly clear lately. I think my eyes were just dry from sitting out in the wind for a week looking for deer. At least I hope that is it.

It was good tonight to get home and see Scarlett. She ran into my arms and it felt good just being a dad. I am more excited about this holiday season than I have been in a long time. Good things are happening.

November 17 Friday Day 36

I pinned both HCG and T while Scarlett was at church last night. Took about 1.5 minutes start to finish. I'm becoming an expert at this. My belly fat was tough again though and the needle kind of popped in after some pressure. It hurt.

And I woke up this morning with no wood at all and drawn up balls. Will I ever make sense of this?

At least I did sleep well for 7 hours and woke up feeling rested. Scarlett and I had a good morning getting her ready for school, and I was just in a pleasant mood all the way around. But where is my wood??!!

I texted Kristi last night to give me a shout when she comes in for the holidays. No response. Will I ever get lucky with women again?

Jewel texted me though. I'll plan to see her in the coming weeks. I am getting performance anxiety just thinking about that sexy woman. But I gotta live my life, man.

The Bronco gets delivered in a couple of hours. I'm stoked about having such a badass manly vehicle. I probably would have been a bit timid driving it around before, but now I feel like just flipping someone the bird if they fuck with me. Ha!

5:10 PM I have felt awesome all day. I worked all morning after taking Scarlett to school, then worked out at noon. It was a good chest day, but my shoulders were bothering me on the press so I had to use abbreviated form and go very slow. I did my bands last night. I will incorporate stretching back into my routine to keep those shoulders healthy. No more surgeries if I can help it.

I found the bitchy young blonde who rarely looks my way kind of checking me out today. She works in the adjoining gift shop and sometimes walks over through the gym. Today she walked by like 5 times. She can't be more than about 24, but I swear she was trying to get my attention. There was only an older couple there besides me, so no reason for her to be walking back and forth through the gym. In the past, she was bitchy to Scarlett and kind of snooty so I've never talked to her. Should I now? She is thin as a rail. Her ass is maybe 12" across. I could have some fun with that.

When I got home the Bronco was delivered. It's a damn beast. Needs some work but nothing major. Most immediate items are the steering, brakes, and hubs. After that the doors need new hinges because they sag. This will be a fun project. I cruised around town with Scarlett and it is damn difficult to drive, but I'll never admit that to all the people who call me a dumbass for buying an old 4x4. They can suck it. I'm a man now. I have a Bronco.

So I've been off the Trintellix since Tuesday now and I feel better. I know that stuff helped get me through the worst of the neurological Lyme, but it also made me feel like nothing was real. It kept the derealization kind of lingering around. I already feel more like an improved version of my old self. I am damn happy to be off antidepressants. I pray I never need them again.

My balls have hung pretty well today after being kind of tight this morning. And I have had great energy. I thought I would need a nap, but I have just been a busy bee all day.

I weighed 188 at the gym. WTF?? I gained 3 lbs. while hunting for 5 days? I am DETERMINED to trim down. My goal is under 180 by year end, then down to 175 by Valentine's. I think that is an attainable and worthy goal. I expect to add some lean muscle mass even as I cut since my T will be high for the first time since a teenager. So I know I won't lose a ton of weight and get all skinny as long as I'm lifting and eating decent. But Damnit, I will not get any heavier. I have not weighed this much in close to 6 years. No way will I go back to fat Rowdy. I have counted my calories today on MyFitnessPal and I am at 1000 so far. That leaves me plenty of room on a lift day to get around 2000 calories or more. I'll be aiming for 1500 net on non-lift days, so I can use some cardio to help me get a deficit. Time to start pounding pavement again and get my ass to running. My caloric intake is actually quite low for a man, but I just know that is where my requirements are right now. Perhaps they will rise over time.

9:42 PM I had a hell of a mood swing this evening, but it seems to have passed. We went to eat with my parents and on the way back my head began to hurt and I got real foggy. Then the girls started asking to go skating and asking to go to Walmart and I got aggravated and had to refrain from blowing up. The girls got mad at me for not giving in to their requests and stormed off, and I sat in silence for a bit and let it pass. I'm all better now, but I'll keep an eye on those. Lyme or hormones or middle-aged frustration?

11/18 Saturday Day 37
My balls were drawn up high and tight this morning. Very tight. I slept fitfully and woke up feeling a little depressed. I am wondering if it is the fatigue from such a long deer hunt combined with going off the antidepressants or some Lyme creeping back.

The morning was kind of foggy and I was able to shake off the depression. I feel better now. Just a little cold and chilly. I definitely want to get my thyroid numbers drawn again.

I have noticed some body acne on my chest and a couple of pimples on my cheeks. I have not had face pimples in a long time other than the occasional small whitehead. These are pretty big ones. Not cool.

The chest acne is in part due to wearing sweaty Under Armour base layer for 5 days hunting. I am using some Proactive Body Wash to get it to clear up.

I feel the urge to snack right now even though I had a good lunch of baked chicken and deer chili. A protein cookie would be tasty. Or pumpkin pie. Either one.

Never heard back from Kristi. Bummer. We kind of hooked up at a party once my senior year in high school, but I did not finish job. I was hoping for another shot at that. Maybe she'll be home for Christmas and look me up.

I don't feel like going to the gym but I think I'd feel better afterward. Even if I just go and walk/jog for a while. Maybe do some abs. Since I lifted yesterday I will not lift today. That's my policy. But some light cardio could only help my mood. Maybe after my nap...

5 PM Quick update. After lying in the recliner watching football for an hour, my balls have elected to descend and hang as low as ever. Nice and full and warm, just like they should be. I salute them. I just wish they would stick around for a while.

11/19 Sunday Day 38
I woke up feeling better this morning. My mind was clear and my mood was excellent. No morning wood though. I am very curious to see where my numbers are. I seem to have hit a sweet spot at some point but have ventured out of that zone.

During Sunday school at church I was very much in command of my thoughts. I expressed myself clearly and boldly and the students took note. Not like I used to be where I might fumble for the words and come off sounding weak. I had something to say and I said it and that was it. I enjoyed it.

After that Scarlett and I worked on the Bronco. I managed to replace the old original locking hubs with some Mile Marker stainless steel ones. At first I ran into some trouble and could feel the frustration rising like it always did, but I backed away and thought about it and did some more research on the internet, and when I returned to the task everything fit together pretty nicely. We drove the Bronco to the gym and it rode fine. I got some nice compliments from two young dudes on how badass the rig is. Would have been better if it was two young hotties but you gotta start somewhere.

Lexi was the only one in there. She's hot in a slutty kind of way and very young - maybe 21. We exchanged pleasantries as always and that was about it, but I caught her sneaking peeks at me on occasion. I think she is mostly checking to see if I am checking her out, which I am careful not to do until I can feel her looking my way. She has a boyfriend and is 21 years younger, so it's a longshot. But as Jim Carey says, "So you're telling me there's a chance."

I performed a very intense leg workout and could feel the pump in my quads afterward. That is a good feeling, but one I will probably pay for in a day or two. I weighed in at 187.4, so down a pound. And that is after a large lunch following the church service and some protein cookies for snacks before we went. Below 180 by Christmas - that is my goal. I can do it.

11/20 Monday Day 39
I had morning wood today! It only lasted until I got up to pee, but it was there in all its rock hard glory. Nice to see it again.

And my boys are hanging decent today. Perhaps they just needed to adjust to a new normal and could not decide what to do or where to go. Either way I appreciate them making an appearance.

My mind was calmer and clearer this morning. I simply got up, got ready for work, got Scarlett up, made some coffee, and began my day of kicking ass. Now I am at the office feeling solid as a rock and looking forward to knocking some shit out today. It is Thanksgiving week so a lot of my colleagues are off, but I have some catching up to do from the deer hunt so I am working half days.

I have committed to a 24 hour fast today. Having read Brad Pylon's "Eat Stop Eat", and performed many cleansing fasts in the past, I know first-hand the power they have to improve digestion and kick start fat loss. I always have good energy on fasting days, and this day will be no exception. I am excited about the challenge!

10:26 PM No fap November did not last. I got kind of horny this evening before I left to go to the gym, and rather than suffer through watching Lexi in her yoga pants, I elected to call November done and fap away. But I was disappointed to discover that I could barely get an erection and could barely maintain it once I did. I even looked at a little porn, which I have not done in months, and it did not seem to help. Shit.

I did have a decent gym session. Since I worked legs yesterday, I just did some ab work tonight then ran a mile. I pushed my pace pretty good and was winded at the end, so I was satisfied with the effort. When I got home my head was all cloudy and it has gotten more so since then. I guess this is some type of brain fog. Likely Lyme related. Will that shit ever subside? It's not uncomfortable. I'm totally relaxed and chilled out. No depression either. But man my focus is just gone. I took an Epsom salt bath and pretty much just zoned out in there. I can barely hold my head up now. I wonder also if it was the fast or if maybe my estradiol is high? I pinned today so I'll wait and get bloods on Wednesday.

I did have good energy during my fast though. Towards the end I hated to even end it. I had a healthy snack of chicken salad, hummus, and Triscuits. And a protein cookie for dessert. Around 800 calories total, so a solid post-fast meal. I look forward to doing this again, unless I can correlate it somehow to my weak erections. Cortisol perhaps? It's been nearly a year since I had the saliva test done. I was sick as hell then and the test still came back near perfect. I suppose it's worth doing again just to make sure. When did life get so freaking complicated? How much I desire to just have a normal sex life with a good woman or two, and to be able to get decent gains in the gym when I bust my ass. All while feeling emotionally balanced and in control. Sometimes that seems so damn far away from where I am. But I persevere, like a damn Koi fish. It's all I know to do.

11/21 Tuesday Day 40
No wood this morning, but my mind was clearer and I felt more positive. I also looked and felt leaner after my fast yesterday. I recall waking up in the middle of the night to pee and I did have nocturnal wood, so that is better than no wood at all.

I feel very calm today. Like I can just glide through my day getting shit done and nothing will through me off balance. I like this feeling of well-being.

Today will be pull day at the gym. Most guys love chest day but I don't due to my shoulders. I love pull day. Lat pulls. Bent over rows. Seated rows. And some curls to torch my biceps. I should take measurements of them now so I can compare in 3 months and again in 6 months. The gun show. Haven't had real guns since my twenties. This will be fun!

I appreciate days like this when my mind is at peace. Too many of them have spent in mental turmoil. In darkness that could find no light. I take solace in knowing I have an inner strength that guides to a better place, no matter how I might arriver there.

11/22 Wednesday Day 41
No wood this morning. None. It's frustrating. Not really horny either. If Megan Fox showed up and said "Let's go", I'd probably ask her to rub my shoulders instead. I have faith though. I know it is a matter of fine tuning and then I'll be chasing women around town with my dick out shaking it at them. Fun times ahead! I also realize I am making too much of this sex issue. Baby steps. I can't really go from sick and tired and celibate to porn star overnight. That just wouldn't be fair. Although I did have occasional sex while I was really sick, so I guess I was never completely without.

I did have a nice workout yesterday. I had sooo forgotten what it's like to get a good pump. My lats, back, and biceps were so engorged that I could barely move my arms around by the end of the workout. That hasn't happened in years. Honestly, I am impressed with my consistency in the gym these past few years while seeing so little results and while being very sick. Even on days where I had no energy and was in so much pain I could barely walk, I would still go to the gym and lift baby weights. Just come curls and some walking to remind myself I was not dead yet. Now I have purpose again when I go in there. I also noticed that weights I have been working with are getting easier, and I can pump out a few more reps even when I think I should be spent. I weighed 186.4, so down a pound or so.

Another positive note is I flirted with Becky at the drugstore when I went to pick up my prescription strength Omega-3 pills. And she flirted back. I sent her a message afterwards and she responded. I'm so brave.

And then later Kristi texted from out of the blue that she still wants to see me. She sent a pic from a beach somewhere. Apparently she took off on vacation with her son. Strange girl, but I've yet to meet a normal one. I'll catch up with her either this weekend or over Christmas.

I am about to get blood work done at the local clinic, then I will review the results next week with my clinic. I have to travel to Richmond, VA on Monday, so it will be next Friday before I review the labs. But I can view them online in a few days and at least see what's going on.

I slept a solid 8 hours last night of uninterrupted sleep, but I was not wide awake when the alarm went off. Just a little groggy. But as soon as I rolled out of bed I shook it off and was ready to go. Again, labs will tell the tale. I swear my eyebrows are thinning out and my hairline is getting higher, but I am trying not to obsess over it. I got a haircut yesterday and showed it to my stylist, so when I get it cut again she can compare. I am sure I am obsessing over nothing.

5:42PM I got my labs drawn. I added in DHEA just for good measure. It was really low back when I sick so I began a supplement to raise it. Being low in that hormone means a weakened immune system besides the hormonal implications, so it was important to be in a good range when fighting Lyme. Last time I checked it was around 300. But I also read that supplementing can cause hair loss. Maybe that is why my eyebrows are half gone rather than low thyroid. And since I read it on the internet I know it must be true.

I pinned HCG this evening. Still lots left in the bottle. I believe it only lasts 60 days and that day is approaching. Memory says I read somewhere that you can preload syringes and freeze them and they will last longer. I am making a mental note to study that further.

One thing I noticed today while having lunch with Scarlett is that my mind is not constantly chattering away like it always has. At first I thought maybe I was kind of zoned out, but then I realized I was perfectly in tune with the present moment. I just wasn't obsessing over every little thing. I never thought about low T contributing to that, but I suppose it is possible. Or maybe my mind just takes little vacations now. Either way I'm good.

10:38PM I drifted off in the recliner for about an hour and woke up at 7:30. Missed dinner at my parents. The 8 hours of solid sleep just doesn't quite last until bedtime right now. It did at first it seems, but not now. Anyway, I got up and went to the gym and walked for 30 minutes. I ran just for a few minutes on a steep incline, then walked the rest of the time. It was pretty relaxing and about all I wanted to do today. I saw a large group of people at the bar next door to the gym and I almost dropped in and had a beer with everyone. I would have never thought of doing that before. I just feel more social right now compared to years past. That's a good thing?

11/23 Thursday Day 42
Thanksgiving is here. I am thankful for how much my mood and emotional well-being has improved, and thankful for the many great erections I have to look forward to along with an improved body composition and overall quality of life.

I have lost some of that kick ass attitude I had the first few weeks. Those weeks being the ones I was taking a double dose. Emotionally I am in a great place. Calm. Relaxed. Anxiety and depression free.

But my motivation has slipped. That drive to get shit done has faded just a bit. I'm allowed a few days off. I will not dwell on it.

No sign of morning erections today. And my boys are high and tight. But I feel pretty damn good overall. I'll take it.

11/24 Friday Day 43
I feel pretty damn good today all things considered. We got in after midnight from watching a football game. Damn opposing team broke our quarterback's ankle.

I slept to around 8 then got up and had some coffee. No morning wood, but I felt good again. Where is my wood? I want my wood! I pinned this morning since we got in so late. Took maybe 1 minute start to finish. No pain. No blood.

My sister is having a party tonight. I messaged Becky about it but have not heard back from her. She would be fun to share my non-erection with. Very tight body. No tits, but very tight.

Overall I ate pretty well on Thanksgiving. Lots of turkey and green beans. Some deviled eggs and sweet potato casserole. I had one small slice of sweet potato pie. That was my only indulgence. At the ballgame I had peanuts and water. And a little whiskey. It was a football game. You are supposed to drink whiskey at those.

I am disappointed to see the chest acne has not cleared up yet. I am using the Proactive on it daily, and maybe it is a little bit better. But it's still there. I might be a little embarrassed about that if it is not gone during my next sexual encounter. It will clear up soon. Does it all ever come together?

Today was chest day in the gym. My shoulders did not hurt as bad when pressing. Still a little bit of impingement, but not as bad as before. I have been using my bands and stretching to strengthen those joints.

I was stronger today. My last set on the bench I was shooting for 230 8 times. I did it 15 times. I have to say I am impressed with the changes in body composition that are now taking form. I thought it would take much longer. I guess since I already had a good habit of lifting that all I needed was a little testosterone and some physical healing to see some results. I weighed in at 185. Down 3.5 lbs. from my max weight a couple of weeks ago. And I look more solid. My quads have a little shape to them now. I have always had such chicken legs - it will be cool to have tree trunk legs if that is possible. Probably not, but adding even a little bit of muscle will most definitely help.

This evening as I was getting ready for my sister's party, I noticed my jeans felt tighter through the butt and thighs. That's a good thing. I've always left the ass of my jeans kind of empty. Maybe if my glutes pop out girls will be checking out my ass. Maybe.

11/25 Saturday Day 44
No wood this morning, but I stayed up way too late. We had a great time at my sister's party, but I could not sleep when I got home. I was just full of energy. Eventually I did drift off after reading about natural remedies for estrogen control. Things like DIM and Calcium D-Glucarate and eating shit tons of broccoli. Or was it two shit tons? Hard to recall.

And while I did not awake with morning wood, a few simple thoughts of Jewel naked got me rock hard in no time. And very engorged again. I could have done some damage if she had been here this morning. And my boys are hanging decent this morning. I can find NO correlation between anything I do and the hanging of my balls. Just some days they hang, some days they don't. Shit.

We are off to see the family soon for another Thanksgiving gathering. I am fasting until we eat at 4pm, then loading up on turkey and vegetables. Skipping dessert this time. I cheated last night when I got in. I was ravenous after my sister's party. Maybe it was the chest workout from earlier, or maybe just empty whiskey belly. But I made two peanut butter and honey sandwiches and ate them before bed. I haven't done shit like that in years. I am not really a late snacker, but damn I was hungry. Next time I'll try and remember to drink a big glass of water instead.

11/26 Sunday Day 45
We've got wood! I woke up with a raging boner and it was magnificent. I only needed someone to shake it at. I stared at it lovingly then washed it thoroughly in the shower.

And on top of that, my balls were still hanging low and full. Gloriously low and full. All is right in the world again.

While Scarlett was getting ready for Sunday school, I pinned my HCG. Took only a minute.

Mentally I was in a good mood, albeit a bit cloudy at times. It's like the cloud is there and then it lifts. Weird.

This afternoon I was worn out for some reason and just wanted to nap, but Scarlett wanted to play so we messed around the house and took our dog to the golf course to run. I wish I had his energy.

I dozed in the recliner after that for maybe 20 minutes, then woke up and found the motivation to get to the gym. Leg day. I pushed good weight on the leg press, then did a tough round of Bulgarian split squats. I like those better. I had a good pump in my quads that I have not had since college. Then I did a full set of leg curls along with nice calve work and I was done. My legs were swollen when I left. It's been a rare occasion that I get a good pump on legs, even back during my heavy squatting days. I could get used to this.

After that we decorated the tree and watched a Hallmark Christmas movie, and I realized I miss true romance. As cheesy as those movies are, it stirred something within that told me I am ready to sweep a woman off her feet. Time to get cracking. Literally.

11/27 Monday Day 47
I woke up with great wood again. The only thing I have changed in the past few days is to quit taking my DHEA supplement. This has resulted in better erections and full hanging balls. What the hell would the relationship be there? I'm not a doctor, but I do stay at a Holiday Inn Express on occasion.

Whatever is going on I want more of it. I flew to Richmond, VA, today and could actually feel my balls against my legs while walking. It has been a good long while since that happened. I did not ogle women in the airport but felt like I could take one on if the chance arose. And I had some anxiety.

On the flight from Memphis to Atlanta, I had just a touch of anxiety after take-off. Not enough to really worry me, but it was there. I was able to let it go and it did not return, even when I fell asleep on the Atlanta to Richmond flight and I woke up suddenly and had to catch my breath. I was immediately calm where in the past I would fight to maintain control. Not sure what to make of it if anything - just an observation.

I feel good right now in the hotel room, but I am ready for bed and it is only 8:30 PM. I slept okay last night, but not great. I have been off ZMA for a while and that always helped my sleep before. Something about the magnesium in it assists with sleep. Plus it has other health benefits, and I like benefits. I'll order some and have it waiting on me when I get home. I wish Jewel was here.

11/28 Tuesday Day 48
I got wired last night once I got in bed and had some trouble drifting off to sleep. Then I slept fitfully as it seemed I could not fall into a deep sleep like I had become accustomed to. I awoke periodically throughout the night feeling a buzzing inside - much like when I was first sick with Lyme. That shit better not be coming back.

No wood when the alarm went off this morning, but I am not surprised with my poor sleep. My boys were still hanging low though, so that was nice to wake up to. I should mention I had a few margaritas at the Mexican place across from the hotel. Perhaps the sugar and alcohol contributed to my sleep issue. I will refrain from that tonight. Just straight whiskey - no sugar.

My mood has been somber so far. I am working at our Richmond, VA plant and even though I have been clear minded and productive, I really feel like saying fuck it to all of this. My drive is just not here right now. I suppose that is something I can control by deliberately bringing it back when it fades, but it would be nice if sustained itself without my effort.

I checked online for my lab results and the T and E levels are not back yet, but the CBC results were. Some interesting observations that would require a hematologist to interpret. Mostly everything was in normal range, but the hematocrit which is the main concern on TRT was low. 41.4 on a scale of 42-52. I suppose that is a good thing as it could only rise the longer I am on TRT, and it also means that being forced to give blood is not in my near future. I know I was diagnosed as iron-deficient anemic last year after my Lyme battle, so perhaps that has not corrected itself.

The other two items that were out of range were mean platelet volume and mean corpuscular hemoglobin concentration which were both just a touch low. I do not know what that means in the grand scheme of things. A quick Google search provides too many possibilities to really point at any one thing. I will discuss with the clinic and see what they say, but none of them were very far out of range so perhaps it doesn't mean anything.

I still take an iron supplement about twice per week, but apparently it is not enough. I will request iron labs to be run again soon and see how that looks. Hopefully the rest of the labs will be in today or tomorrow. I am very curious to see where I stand on the big T scale.

I am tired right now and wish I had better sleep. I am ordering some damn ZMA today so I will have it when I get home.

11/29 Wednesday Day 49
I had decent wood when I woke up this morning. I took some Nyquil last night so I could sleep and it worked. I went to bed around 10 and did not move until 6:15 AM. It was hard to get up though. I felt groggy and just wanted to lie in bed all morning. Need to shake this cold.

Funny thing about having a cold is I have not had one in a few years now. Having Lyme meant such a diminished immune system, so even if I had contact with cold germs or any viruses I usually had no immune response and did not even know I was under further attack. At least now I know my immune system is fighting this crud off.

I texted Jewel yesterday but have not heard back. I am ready to try out my new penis and so I requested a visit with her. I expect a response today.

Looking in the mirror this morning, I see my belly is still soft but a little bit flatter, and my chest and shoulders are more muscular. My legs did not look too different, though I am positive they are filling out some. There is no gym in the hotel so I just walked on the treadmill on a steep incline for 15 minutes last night. Better than nothing. I'll do some pushups tonight and ab work tonight.

My goal is to be under 180 by year end. I am looking forward to weighing in at the gym Thursday when I get home. I am predicting 184-185, which leaves me set up to lose a lb. a week for the month of December. Should work out about right assuming I don't imbibe too much eggnog.

Mentally I am working to get my drive back. I have accepted that it is something I may have to cultivate and not expect it to just be there automatically with the addition of testosterone shots. So I continue to work on visualizing my goals and objectives and expecting my mind to be clear and sharp to help accomplish them. Sounds like a plan.

11/30 Thursday Day 50

No wood this morning, but boys were still hanging low. I have read, I believe on Peak Testosterone site, that the TRTimprovements to the penis can take 6-9 months for full effect. I suppose I'll just keep tracking progress and see what my time frame is.

On a normal week I would have pinned the HCG last night, but I did not want to take it with me on the plane. I could have. I have a nice little kit with ice pack that holds a few preloaded syringes and would have kept one cool until I got to the hotel, but I figured waiting 24 hours would not have a huge effect.

I woke up early to catch my flight, and felt pretty solid even with the head cold. Which is getting progressively worse.

I had zero anxiety on the plane. Much more grounded and calm. I was just coughing a lot which sucked. I know the people around me did not care for it.

I started a new book on the plane ride home that I think will really go along nicely with the new feeling of confidence I am obtaining. It is called Gorilla Mindset by Mike Cernovich. It is basically a book on how to take control of your life. I have read other such books, but this one seems to have a no bullshit flow to it that the other books were missing. This guy seems like a man's man, so to speak.

I went ahead and pinned the HCG this afternoon when I got home. I upped the dose to .5 mL because I read online that is the minimum required to retain intratesticular volume. It was on the internet so it must be true. Is intratesticular a word?

All of my lab results are available now.

Total Test = 697
Free Test = 17
Estradiol = 28
DHEA = 127

Not bad numbers. I suppose I thought total T might be higher, but that was at a trough so those are good numbers. I meet tomorrow with the clinic to review. I am sure they will be pleased.

Also, there is another deep pimple developing on my left cheek. Could get ugly. My chest looks better though.

Friday December 1 Day 51
No wood again. Where has my wood gone? My motivation is zilch. My mood is somber. Borderline sad. I realize as I type this and mark Day 51 of my journey, that I have not had sex once in those 51 days. Unfucking acceptable. I have not had dry spells like this since I began having sex at around 16. Just sad. Makes me sad.

I met with the dude at the Wellness clinic. He likes my numbers but wants the DHEA to come up. But instead of supplementing with that he is checking pregnenolone. He says that is what they use quite often with TRT to supplement other hormones as it is the "master" hormone. Sounds cool. I don't care today.

He checked my thyroid panel also and wants to look at something called reverse T3. I think this guy knows his shit pretty well. My eyebrows are getting wispy and my widow's peak is getting higher. I'll be pissed if I lose hair over this. So far conquering my depression is the only major victory. Anxiety is markedly improved but it was already fading due to the meditations I was doing.

My cold is getting worse. I'm hacking up shit and my head feels like a big marshmallow. Getting sick just blows. I just want to lie in bed all damn evening, but Scarlett's mom has insisted we come over to her house to watch the Christmas parade since she lives right in town. I'm a team player in this co-parenting deal but damn I dislike hanging around her and her friends. At least I can drink some of her new husband's top shelf bourbon.

Saturday December 2 Day 52
How about I just don't even mention wood anymore unless it shows up again. Damnit.

Last night was a low point for me. I took Scarlett to the parade and felt shitty due to the cold. On top of that I was the recipient of lots of sympathy looks from her friends for being the dad who had no better option than to hang out in the shadows of his ex-wife's parade party while she and her friends and their kids had a ball. I hate those fucking looks. People wanting to feel sorry for me.

The bitch of it is I could care less what those fuckers think. I don't need or want their sympathy. Two of the ladies there beside my ex have shared their bodies with me at other points of our lives so I damn sure don't need their sympathy either.

And Becky. She was there looking kind of easy with that toothy grin and Bud Light tallboy in hand. She is interested, and I could tell if I could have separated her from the pack of jackals just for a while I could have made some damn progress with her. But she is best buds with my ex-wife's younger sister, and there is a whore code I'll have a tough time cracking there. So to speak.

Anyway, I had a nice sip of said new husband's Buffalo Trace, enjoyed the parade, then Scarlett and I came home and enjoyed our evening. Today we have had fun at the house with the dog and I got a good lift session in this afternoon. Chest day. On a Saturday. My shoulders screamed a little bit but I powered through. I just limit the range of motion and go slow so as not to do any damage. If I continue to do my stretches and auxiliary work I am sure they will tighten up. I did 250lbs 8 times. Most I have pushed in a long time. And I weighed in at 185.3. I'll be under 180 by Christmas.

Sunday December 3 Day 53

I had morning wood when I first woke before daylight! Not sure what time it was, but I recall waking up and it was hard. I went back to sleep and when I woke up later it was not hard. What does it mean? Who the hell knows?

I do know that my boys seem to be permanently hanging low again. This is a nice development. Perhaps it is because my body temperature has been closer to normal since I have been feeling better. It was 98.8 one day, and 98.6 yesterday. Maybe this cold is a blessing in disguise. My body temperature was really low when I was in the throes of Lyme, and it never felt right to take my temperature and see numbers a couple degrees cooler than normal.

My mood is better today I suppose. I realize I at least have a new set point. Before, I was fighting depression pretty hard and my really bad days were like "keep a gun out of my hand" days. Now an off day is just a blah day with little motivation to kick ass. As long as those are the bottom and not the norm, I will be pretty pleased with that development.

After church I just felt beat down from this freaking cold, so I napped for about 3 hours in the recliner. It was glorious. Just what I needed. I suppose I should share that I had some kind of weird sex dream that seemed to be American Pie related. Shit. This dry spell is warping my brain.

After that it was nearly dark out, so I went to the gym and just walked on an incline for an hour. I even worked up a sweat. It was a good walk.

Gave me time to get my head right about some things. Like not obsessing over lack of sex, focusing on my business opportunities, and mastering my emotions. Good stuff.

After that I went to Walmart to pick up some stuff and ran into my neighbor Nicole. She has acted a little uncomfortable around me the last few times I have seen her. What's up with that? At first I wasn't sure but tonight I could swear she was turned on by my presence and it made her nervous around me. I've known this girl all her life, and her husband is a friend of mine, so this is a new development if so. Her husband is kind of a girly man. But even if she is turned on by me, I am not looking to get it on with another man's wife. Not my style no matter how long this dry spell lasts.

I heard from Jewel today. I am guaranteed sex for New Year's Eve, so that should relieve some pressure. We are going either to New Orleans or to Jacksonville, Florida to watch MSU in the Gator Bowl. I'm down for either. Or she could come here and we'll watch the game naked in the whirlpool tub. Any of those options suit me just fine.

December 4 Monday Day 54
We have wood! I woke up with a nice surprise this morning. Nice and full and ready to hammer nails. You know what was different about last night? No alcohol. I had not put that together until now. I drank every night in Richmond because I had dinner with a colleague, and I drank Friday and Saturday night because it was the weekend and I had a cold.

But not last night. I just got in bed around midnight and instantly fell asleep. And when I woke up around 7:30am all was right in the world. I was a bit groggy though. Like I could have slept all morning.

I am hoping it is just this damn head cold, but I took a 3 hour nap yesterday afternoon, slept over 7 hours last night, and woke up tired. I then worked all morning until noon, got in the recliner and drifted off for another 2 hours. I appreciate the sleep but damn I've got shit to do.

This evening I completed a very nice leg workout. They were rubbery when I got done - the way they should be. I have had a hard time pushing them to that point these past several years. My knees groaned a little, but I was careful with them and used good form.

My mood was odd when I got to the gym. Like I was floating in a cloud. It wasn't positive or negative - just there. It took me a while to put my finger on what it was, but I think I figured it out. A COMPLETE LACK OF FEAR. I realized at some point in my workout that I was not really afraid of anything. Not death, failure, rejection, illness, financial woes, women. Not really anything. It was surreal.

One thing the past couple of years dealing with Lyme taught me is that my life was driven by fear for the most part (thanks mom). I lived with obsessive thoughts and let my inner child bully me into safe spaces. All was quiet this evening at the gym. It's like a new baseline. One from where I am free to go anywhere. I shall ponder more on this as I work my way through Gorilla Mindset.

December 5 Tuesday Day 55

Wood again today! I initially woke up around 6 AM with no wood, but fell back asleep as I did not have to be up until 7. When I woke up at 7 there was wood. Not quite as massive as I would like, but I'll take it. Still no consistency here. Weird. I will say that as I dressed last night in my closet to hit the gym, for some reason I stood there and pictured the cute redhead at the medical clinic giving me a hummer. Random sex thoughts have not been part of my life in quite a while. I was hard in no time, and fully engorged. So that was fun.

This morning I woke up with a sense of purpose. I stayed up later than I would like. It was after midnight before I finally fell asleep, and I know I woke a few times during the night for different reasons.

But I woke up ready to get shit done. No more excuses. Focused on today's tasks and what can move me closer to my goals. Namely an abundant dating life and financial freedom.

4:40 PM I have been super productive today at the office. I was absolutely on point during a 2 hour meeting with outside consultants, and every interaction today I felt completely in control of. Now it is time to go and get my daughter and spend quality time with her. I am loving this crystal clear focus and feeling of purpose. This is a new me.

December 6 Wednesday Day 56

So-so wood today. Not completely hard, but not flaccid. Perhaps I am beginning to obsess over this, but one of the things I looked forward to was waking in the mornings with a good old boner staring at me like I had in the days of my youth. Perhaps I should just be happy when it does occur and not give it a thought when it does not. Perhaps.

I woke kind of foggy but got out of bed and got going. I felt cold. Really cold. The house was cold so maybe that was part of it, but not all of it. When I got to work my hands were so cold I could barely write. This used to happen when I was on a very strict intermittent fasting regimen and was disciplined in my daily routine. I had not noticed it as much during my recent fasting trial until today. Maybe I am finally beginning to drop some fat?

I weighed in at the gym tonight at 186.4. Disappointing, but even though the weight is not changing I feel my body is. I just feel more muscular and like I am filling out my shirts and pants better. I think my face has leaned up a bit, but the belly fat not so much. Maybe I am going through more of a "recomp" rather than a cut. If a "recomp" truly exists. I would say I am consistently under or right at 2000 calories a day. Combined with strength training that should allow me to drop some fat. But that damn scale is sure stuck around 186. I hate to cut calories much more, but I could try 1700 as a goal and see what happens. With higher test levels I should maintain most of my muscle even on a caloric deficit such as that.

My mind was clear most of the day, and when it seemed to drift I practiced the presence exercises as described in Gorilla Mindset. Very helpful in bringing me back to the here and now. But as I truly check in with my body it is easy to feel that I am not 100% yet. Whether it is lingering Lyme, a slow thyroid, needing more time to dial in my T regimen, or a little of all of them - I know I am not optimal.

Part of that frustrates me and sends just a wrinkle of fear that I may never feel 100%, and part of me is excited that at age 42 I have a chance to continue to feel better while most my age continue to feel worse from here on out. I choose excitement.

This morning I blew up at Scarlett and yelled at her because she would not choose a coat and get in the car. She was making us late by piddling around and it just crawled all over me. My yelling made her cry, which then made me feel worse. I am mindful of what happened though and feel I can harness that frustration and redirect it next time. Yelling at my daughter is out of character for me. I do not intend to do so again.

STARTING TO SEE SOME BETTER DAYS

December 7 Thursday Day 57

I slept 7 solid hours and woke up before the alarm went off at 5:58 AM. I literally opened my eyes and my mind began working on today's tasks, then I stopped and said to myself, "Self, wait a damn minute. What time is it?" This prompted me to look at my iPhone and see that I had about 5 minutes until the alarm went off. All good.

I could feel what I assume was cortisol flowing through my veins. It kind of gave me a buzz. It was a touch uncomfortable at first, but I relaxed into it and did some deep breathing and felt better. I did a 10 minute meditation on my goals, then rolled out of bed and started getting shit done. Zero wood. Balls riding high. Whatever.

My mind is totally calm and clear this morning. Could be because I rubbed one out after running some errands. I am not going to beat myself up for it. No sex recently means I need an outlet. Once every couple of weeks is by no means excessive. And I felt calmer afterwards. Although it was concerning that my erection was weak, my orgasm was also quick and weak, and my load was light and watery. Certainly not adult film star worthy. Perhaps the pipes were just rusty.

I know I am spending New Year's Eve with Jewel and will have a sex marathon, and I could possibly see Kristi between now and then. 2018 will be a year with more sex, Damnit. I miss that part of my life.

My face and chest are much clearer now. Actually my skin looks better overall I'd say. That chest breakout was scary, but it did not last. Not sure about the two big pimples that showed up on my face. Very deep. Don't want to see any more of those.

I did my biweekly pin this evening of test. .25 mL in the right shoulder. No blood. It did sting a bit. It's weird how sometimes I don't even feel the needle, and others it feels like a wasp stinging me. Tonight was a wasp.

I walked for an hour at the gym. Midway I jogged for nearly a mile, then resumed walking. I felt shin splints coming on. I would very much like to jog more consistently. I ran no races this year after feeling so sure I would once I beat Lyme disease. Hell I could barely walk a year ago. I have allowed myself to take for granted the gift of health I was given. No more. I shall run a race and run it soon, even if it is only against myself.

12/8 Friday Day 58

I woke up feeling like a damn boss today. No snooze. I slept solid until the alarm went off, awoke and said a prayer, made my bed, and let the dog out.

After that I visualized a goal I am working on, then made coffee and wrote some affirmations. After that I took a cold shower which took my breath away and made me scream like a bitch, then I shivered through getting dressed and was out the door to the office, ready to kick some ass.

And I had half a boner when I woke up that lasted until I drank my coffee. Cool. Boys hanging nicely until the cold shower. They came back down around 11 AM. My book Gorilla Mindset recommends these, but I am not so sure after today. Maybe when it is not 29 degrees outside. Or maybe freaking never again.

At work I have been knocking out one task after another, and putting out fires as they come up. I flirted at lunch with the cute little check out girl at the market, and she made the person behind me wait so she could finish telling me a story. I quite possibly could have mounted her right then and there. I was feeling "on". Or at the very least I feel I could have gotten a discount on a can of soup.

Now it is almost time to pick up Scarlett, and I have this nervous energy running through my veins that screams "don't fuck with me".

The world is real and clear and feels like mine for the taking. Have I ever felt this confident?

No depression. No anxiety. No derealization.

The only thing in the world I could even complain about right now is the pesky ringing in my left ear. But it doesn't bother me. Just a reminder that I am alive.

I look forward to crushing it at the gym this evening, then getting more work done at home later on. I need 2000 words on the Lyme book and some progress on my other projects. No problem.

12/9 Saturday Day 59
I did not crush it at the gym last night. I somehow got sidetracked by going out to eat with my parents. During which time I had a couple of beers. No biggie. But after that I went to their house and proceeded to drink about 5 good whiskey drinks from my dad's cabinet. That was not in my plans.

Yet I woke up with great wood this morning. I mean I really could have laid some damn pipe. And my hangover was barely noticeable. Seems like I should pay a bigger price for such a night. Is high testosterone a miracle hangover cure?

Scarlett and I spent the day at the mall in Florence, AL. I felt pretty alpha walking around and noticed attractive women everywhere we went. Have they always been there? Doesn't seem so, but my radar just picks them up now. Weird. Fun.

An interesting event happened while we were in Target. Scarlett had left the lights on when she was messing around with the switches earlier, so the battery was dead when we got out to the car. In the past I probably would have handled it poorly and got on to her pretty rough, but instead I told her to sit tight. I walked back into Target, purchased some jumper cables, and walked back to the car. I knew what would happen when I popped the hood and hooked up the cables. A dude came along and asked if I needed a jump, to which I replied I did. He pulled his car over and we hooked up and got the car started. I thanked him and he went on his way. I got to walk Scarlett through each step of the interaction, starting with how one should not get upset when things happen. Instead it is wise to immediately assess the situation and focus on a solution. She apologized for the error on her part and I told her no apology necessary because she did not do anything intentionally wrong. She just did not know any better and now she did. And now I have a set of jumper cables in the trunk the way any man should. Or woman. It was a good interaction with a positive result.

Tonight one of my side businesses had a Christmas party uptown. It was a small crowd and one of the clients in attendance is a former fling of mine from years ago. And she looked damn good. I could tell she was kind of checking me out, and if she was not currently married it probably would have been on. But as it was I enjoyed a nice evening feeling very sociable and happy to be out being seen in town. That would not have been the case a few months ago. I would have made an excuse not to go because I would be obsessing over the fact that I would be going alone and would have to talk to people all night. This is much better.

12/10 Sunday Day 60
I am officially 60 days in! Whohoo! The main changes to date are emotional. I'd like to say my sex life has improved, but I would need to have sex to actually gauge that. I'm still a little scared of it honestly. Maybe a lot scared.

At church this morning I felt so calm and present. I kept waiting for my mind to take off the way it used to and spin out of control, but it was perfectly content to just be there.

Afterward I ate a big lunch at mom and dad's, then we drove the old Bronco out to see a friend. It was a nice afternoon and I have not wanted a nap once. I also did not get to the gym at all this weekend which is disappointing, but it is what it is. I'll be in Dallas this week so hopefully the hotel has a decent gym.

12/11 Monday Day 61
I slept so well last night. I mean my eyes closed and then the alarm went off. I might have gotten up once to pee but it could have been a dream. And decent wood when I awoke this morning.

The battery was dead on the car when we tried to leave for school, but instead of getting mad I just hooked up the battery charger to it and told Scarlett to get in the Bronco. So I started that old cold beast up and drove her to school in it without a care in the world.

Then I came back and cranked the car and put my bags in it and drove to Memphis to the airport. I felt like a million bucks all the way there. Totally relaxed and clear minded.

But when I got to the gate I had just a touch of anxiety show up. I faltered a bit getting on the plane, but settled down and relaxed into the flight. I fell asleep about halfway to Atlanta and woke up feeling like I had stopped breathing. It put me in a bit of a panic and it took a few seconds for me to get my breathing regulated. Then I was fine.

I felt great again in Atlanta but once I got to the gate for my connecting flight to Dallas, the anxiety came back up. It pissed me off that it showed up after all this time, and even though I felt like I wanted to be anywhere but on that damn plane, I took a breath and commanded control of my emotions and boarded and took my seat. I was still shaky up until takeoff, then my body seemed to accept that I was in control and it released the anxiety. It's nearly 11 in my hotel and I have not felt a bit of anxiety since.

In fact, I felt very much "on" during dinner with colleagues. And if my young colleague from Atlanta was not in a serious relationship I feel certain I could have her here in the room right now.

The clinic called today and said my thyroid looked good but my pregnenolone was low. So they are calling me in a prescription at a compounding pharmacy to begin supplementation. It will include some DHEA as well. I expect nothing but more good things from this. I have read anecdotal reports on this stuff increasing mood and libido. Nothing wrong with that.

Kristi texted me tonight. We are going out over Christmas. I wonder if she is really a true blonde.

12/12 Tuesday Day 62
I woke up before the alarm this morning and meditated. No wood. So what? I felt good at first, but it did not last.

We left the hotel at 7:15 and I skipped breakfast, then had just coffee at our meeting. After about I'm here in Dallas all week, which is a town I love very much. I could easily live here, and almost did at one point in my youth.

After about an hour of our meeting I felt a wave of depression wash over me. It was weird. Just a feeling that nothing is going right and no matter what I do I'll die and it won't have mattered.

But I was able to take control of my emotions by noon and right the ship. In the past I would have been dominated all day - maybe for days before I snapped out of it. But this time I felt strong enough to change my thoughts and my outlook began to change as well. It was a powerful feeling to realize that even depression has no hold over me now.

After our meetings, we came back to the hotel. I meditated for 15 minutes then did a nice leg workout in the hotel gym. I felt strong but my boys were riding high and tight. Why is that? Hernia? I know it caused that on the left one before. The doctor explained that what was torn was the sheath that covered the cord that leads down to my testicle. Any damage in there and the testicle retracts to protect itself. At one time I thought maybe I had something related to those guys who took Propecia and now experience all kinds of damn issues with their sex parts. The stories on the internet are horrific. My issues are something different. I know when I got the hernia repaired in March of 2017 my boys hung nice and low for a good long while, then slowly pulled back up. My damn balls. I'm just glad I still have them I guess.

At dinner tonight I felt myself flowing in and out of the conversation. I did not feel as alpha as I did last night. There was a large group of at-tractive women at the table next to us drinking and laughing and I found myself wishing I knew what to say to them. Maybe soon I will.

Kate flirted all night as we drank wine, and towards the end of dinner she asked me to come wake her up in the morning and told me what room number she is in. It totally flew over my head and I just joked it away. It wasn't until the drive home that I realized she actually gave me her room number. Girls don't just do that shit randomly. But she lives with her boyfriend and is a colleague so I am not acting on it. Even though I would love to see that big old round booty up in the air. But at least it is progress. I did feel like the hot waitresses in the bar were giving me more looks than I would normally get. I was just carrying myself more confidently and I guess it showed. I also got quite a look from a woman at the bar while we were waiting to be seated. Progress.

We had a group pic made and I feel like I look bloated in it. My skin tone is actually better. A bit deeper and oilier instead of pasty and dry the way I was looking over the past few years. But my face definitely had some roundness to it. It is imperative that I drop these extra pounds and lean out. I might then just be unstoppable.

12/13 Wednesday Day 63
I woke up at 4:26 AM wide awake and with some anxiety. Nothing specific, just a generalized feeling of uneasiness. I did have a great erection so I was pretty proud of that, but it did not last once I woke up good. I tried to go back to sleep. I relaxed my body. Cleared my mind. Prayed.

I went to YouTube and did a guided meditation on releasing anxiety. I felt better but could not sleep, so I ended up hitting the gym and doing a 15 minute HIIT session. After that the anxiety was mostly gone.

A cold shower would have been too much I think, so I took a warm one and then turned it to cool at the end. It felt good.

So I am wondering if something is bothering me that caused the anxiety and sleeplessness. Are my hormones out of balance a bit, did the 3 glasses of wine I drank last night wear off about that time, or something I have not even thought of? Maybe all of the above.

Either way, I am sitting here in the conference room waiting for our meeting to start, sipping coffee and feeling pretty okay now. I think the prayer helped as much as anything. Just haven't talked to God enough lately.

The compounding pharmacy called yesterday and said they will have my pregnenolone/DHEA scrip ready Friday when I get back. I look forward to giving it a try. Even though I have not had sex in a while, I can just tell that my libido is pretty low right now. Just a lack of feeling. Maybe this will help. Maybe I am still scared to try.

8:06 PM I feel better now. When I got back to the hotel I was just spent. I napped for about 30 minutes and woke up in a fog. I lie in bed kind of feeling sorry for myself for feeling so damn crappy and wuss like. Then I pulled my shit together and hit the hotel gym and had a nice chest work-out. After that I was focused and emotionally centered.

I am wondering if my HCG has lost some of its potency. My last shot was Sunday morning and that was at the 60 day mark. My boys are definitely drawing up this week and not hanging full like they have at times. When I get back I'll get a new bottle and make an assessment of the new batch.

For now though all is well. Jewel texted me to confirm our New Year's Eve plans. Only a few more weeks to my sex debut on TRT! Will it be epic or a major fail? Shit I wish I knew. I'm scared.

12/14 Thursday Day 64
Tough start today but it ended okay. I woke up early again around 3 AM feeling wired but tired. I was able to drift back off this time but felt anxious as hell. I did have nice nocturnal wood though.

I woke up again with the alarm around 6:30 exhausted, anxious, and feeling a bit depressed - but with damn good wood. I am hopeful that eventually all the good stuff happens at the same time?

I suffered through the early morning meetings, then I had to give about an hour long presentation. I was surprisingly focused and confident and actually got a small ovation when I was finished. Not too shabby.

But for the rest of most of the day I sat at the conference table wrestling depression and feeling cold. My body just could not seem to warm up.

By the end of the day I seemed to have won the battle with my thoughts, but my body just felt puny and cold. When I got back to the hotel I turned up the heat and lie on the bed for about an hour drifting in and out of sleep.

I got up around 7 and instead of going to the gym I just went downstairs and had dinner and a glass of red wine. I felt better after that. I was too physically beat to exercise. Now my body seems to have regulated its temperature, my mood is not blissful but rather calm and steady, and I am ready for a good night's sleep. That is about all for today.

12/15 Friday Day 65
I woke up at 4:30 AM to catch a flight out of Dallas. No wood. Mood was better though. I expected to have anxiety all the way to the airport but it never came. It was a smooth flight to Atlanta and I enjoyed the time to myself.

I felt confident walking through the airport. Not sure what it was, just a feeling of being okay. I think I even had a few women looking my way just by walking with confidence and purpose with a smile on my face. Maybe.

My mood has certainly been a roller coaster on this trip. I am happy to be home.

12/16 Saturday Day 66
I woke up at 4:30AM this morning to go deer hunting with my father. I wanted to stay in bed, but once I got up and going it was not so bad. It was too early to even tell if I had wood or not. Maybe I did. I found myself thinking about having sex with Jewel while sitting in the deer stand. Damn New Year's Eve cannot get here soon enough.

I dozed off and on in the shooting house and felt totally relaxed. It was some good time spent thinking about 2017 and what I want to accomplish in 2018. I am trying to limit it to a few key items that are achievable. I have been guilty in the past of making a goals sheet with 30+ items on there and just getting overwhelmed. So next year I will be smarter and conquer more goals.

The past few weeks I had really been feeling outgoing and not so caught up inside my head, but at the deer camp I found myself getting quiet and mostly having inner dialogue instead of talking with dad. Maybe it is hormones or maybe it is just that I always argue more with him inside my head than in actual conversation. Perhaps I will eventually develop enough confidence to express my feelings to even my hardass dad.

12/17 Sunday Day 67
We woke up at 4:30 but it was pouring down rain. Thank goodness. That meant we killed the alarm and went back to sleep. I had decent wood lying in my sleeping bag. I was giddy that it was there and gripped it like a little kid would a piece of candy.

We decided not to hunt at all and just packed up and drove home. I was quiet for some reason. My mood was solid - no anxiety or depression. But I was mostly talking inside my head again. I suppose Gorilla Mindset would take control of that and let it out. But I am not there yet. More of a screech monkey mindset right now.

We had Scarlett's Christmas program at church tonight and it was pretty cool. I felt clear minded and very present during the show. I was talkative and friendly with those around me. And Pamela looked at me like I was a different person. Pamela being the hot blonde who lives in Memphis who comes back home on occasion to go to church with her parents.

We are always friendly. I have made some lame attempts at flirting over the past few years. But mostly I feel weak and nervous and beta around her. Or at least I did. Tonight I was all smiles and even patted her arm when I sat down and said hello. She stared me in the eyes with this confused look like she did not even know who I was. I could not tell if it was a good thing or bad. Or neither. But it was different. She did not smile. Just a serious look like she was thinking something she could not share.

I know she has a boyfriend. A doughy looking older fellow that she plays tennis with. The kind of guy who has to be wondering how the hell he pulled a girl like Pamela. This is something to keep an eye on. Stay tuned for future developments.

12/18 Monday Day 68
I woke up early feeling ready to roll. Decent wood. Good mood.

After dropping Scarlett off at school, I drove an hour to visit with my therapist. It was a good session and I was able to recognize how much progress I have made. I think she also recognized how much my mood has improved lately. But I have not discussed TRT with her. Why is that? Maybe next visit.

After that, I got kind of frustrated later in the morning as I finished getting our things ready to leave for Gatlinburg. It seemed the world was against me and all these little things kept popping up impeding our exit.

But I was able to successfully get everything done and pick Scarlett up and we had a nice 6 hour drive to the Smoky Mountains. I felt no anxiety on the drive up. None. I can recall past trips where it was hell navigating the interstate while trying to control my breathing and not freak the fuck out.

This drive was easy breezy. We arrived and our friends the Boyds were already settled in. I had a couple of glasses of red wine and now I am hitting the sack. I feel good about this trip.

12/19 Tuesday Day 69
What wood this morning! It was like being a teenager again. Man I could get used to this. It was there when I woke up before dawn to pee, and again when I woke up about 8. And I mean hard. Damn I wish Jewel or someone else was here to share it with.

We hiked about a 4.5 mile round trip trek up a decent sized mountain to a place called Alum Cave. I elected to fast until after the hike so I skipped breakfast. I had good energy but my mind was foggy. There were moments of clarity, but mostly I felt some of that old derealization where nothing about the moment seemed like it was actually happening. More like viewing the world through virtual reality goggles. It pissed me off at first, but when we got to our summit and chilled, I allowed myself to enjoy the views even if they might not have seemed real.

After that, we went into town and had a late lunch at the Smoky Mountain Brewery. I felt like I had earned a beer so I had 3. And a cheeseburger. I had a side order of broccoli to balance things out. It was all delicious. My mood was positive and I enjoyed being with my daughter and our friends. I flirted a bit with our waitress and she reciprocated.

I was foggy while we watched the girls ice skate. I zoned out a few times and found myself inside my mind again. Time to take control of that and get out of there. Life is happening on the outside.

12/20 Wednesday Day 70
I could have driven nails this morning. I woke up once to pee at 6 AM and could have driven nails then, then slept until 9 AM and woke up at full attention. It was awesome. This is the sweet spot.

My mood is much better today also. Yesterday I was fighting the fog most of the day. Even during our hike up to Alum Cave my mind seemed to be wrestling with itself. But today I felt positive all day. I pinned Monday around noon before we left, so I am past the peak but must be in a good spot before my next pin. Normally I would pin HCG this evening but again I did not want the hassle of travelling with it so I left it at home. I am not sure it makes a lot of difference.

I had nice energy all day and was able to just enjoy being present with my daughter and our friends. We played a game called MagicQuest at Pigeon Forge that required quite a bit of deductive reasoning, and my mind felt sharp.

I also noticed the attractive women there but did not feel that urge deep inside. Although my mood is positive and I am getting good nocturnal and morning wood, my libido appears to be a bit low right now. Perhaps the pregnenolone will help with that some. I am still not having sex so it does not matter much anyway.

I really thought I would have been more motivated to pursue opportunities at this point, but it just has not happened. Maybe after the first of the year.

12/21 Thursday Day 71

Woke up in a bit of a fog this morning. My mood was okay, but my mind was just foggy. Damnit. I could have slept all day probably.

But I got up and had coffee and we went skiing. Once I got going I was surprised at how strong my legs felt and how much energy I was able to tap into. I have not skied since college - some twenty plus years ago. Yet I was able to pick it right up and cut down the mountain with strong legs and core. It felt good. I actually felt kind of athletic, which has not been the case since about the same time ago in college.

I also discovered <u>why</u> my vision gets blurry sometimes and <u>why</u> the world I look at appears a bit distorted. This was one of the scariest symptoms of Lyme disease and I could never figure out quite what caused it. But today while gliding down a slope, I noticed with the all-white background hundreds of floaters and little squiggly lines in my vision. At first I was thinking "what the hell?", but then I was instantly okay with it because it explained so much. There are quite common with people who suffer from late stage Lyme disease. And it let me know I still have a bit of healing to do. This is good news because it means I have not yet reached peak health. That better days are still to come.

It has been a nice mini-vacation. I have felt strong and had good energy. A little bit foggy at times, but no anxiety. I might have felt a touch of depression but not enough to worry that it is settling back in. Overall I am excited about the future. That is a good feeling.

12/22 Friday Day 72

I woke up a bit tired from staying up too late. Don't even remember if I had wood. Probably so. We drove from Gatlinburg to home in 6 hours. Maybe a bit under. That is good time. Scarlett slept a lot of it and I just focused on the road and thought about 2018 and all that might happen.

This is a much better place than last year. Hell last year I was not sure if I would live much longer. I was sure my heart would give out from the strain of being so sick for so many days in a row. My body felt like it weighed

300 lbs. and my breathing was labored even when sitting down. I NEVER want to go back to that. Ever.

Long drives once gave me a bit of anxiety. If I focused too much on reality and being in the moment I would feel a bit of panic and have to distract myself. That was a much shittier way to be than I ever realized at the time. This drive was peaceful. I could focus fully on the moment and take nice deep breaths and know that everything was okay.

I dropped Scarlett off at her mom's then I came home and unloaded. I had good intentions of going to the gym but I was physically beat. I took a nap in the recliner then got up and cleaned house for a while. Now I am ready for to sleep again. Tomorrow is a new day.

12/23 Saturday Day 73
I really blew my diet while in Gatlinburg. Too many beers and apple ciders. Oh well. It's the damn holidays and I am not beating myself up too much. I have total faith that my body is headed in the right direction, even if I feel soft this morning.

My mind is clearing up a bit. I had gotten caught up inside my own head again while in Gatlinburg and did not even realize it. Now I feel more outwardly expressive if that makes sense. My mood is strong and I want to socialize. I have a longing to be with people which is weird for me. I've always been more comfortable alone.

We had a fish fry at my parent's house with all of dad's side of the family. It was a blast and I really felt "on". I was cracking jokes. Picking on younger cousins whom I have rarely engaged in the past, and overall was the center of conversation for much of the day. This was a complete 180 from most of our family gatherings over the past 3 decades. Ones where I sat brooding by myself counting the seconds until it was over. This was damn fun.

This evening I was bored as hell and wanted to go out. Anywhere. It pissed me off that I have no friends who want to do anything and no woman right now close by to hang with. This shit has GOT to fucking change. I can feel my youth dripping away like a leaky faucet.

So I went to the gym and did a high volume low weight leg workout. Something similar to the DTP by Kris Gethrin. I'll pay for it in 2 days but I just wanted to have pumped and rubbery legs. And they feel great.

12/24 Sunday Day 74

Christmas Eve is here. I had excellent nocturnal and morning wood to start my day. I made it to Sunday School and church and then finished my Christmas shopping afterwards. And the most interesting thing happened at the Walmarts that I feel compelled to write about.

I was perusing the kid's aisle when I caught sight of an attractive raven haired woman whom I have never seen before. I smiled a big smile and she returned one even bigger. I got a little spring in my step and continued my shopping, then ran into Hope Williams - a girl I grew up with. Hope still looked good even with a few pounds on her, and we hugged and chatted away about not having shit to do in our small Mississippi town. She went on and on about how good I looked. Weird since I consider myself at least 10 lbs. overweight and I just spent 2 years battling a hellish disease that has left fatigue in my eyes. But she seemed to mean it. Then the raven walked by us and smiled again. Long black hair. Slender body. Dressed nice. Hope and I agreed to find something to do in Iuka soon. I forgot to ask if she is still married. Then I turned back to the kid's aisle to select my gift and get out of there. The raven was standing right where I needed to go. "What the hell?" I thought.

I walked past and said hello to her and joked that I promised I was not following her around. She laughed and we made small talk and it was going great. I joked that since she was following me around she had to help me select a gift for a young girl and she readily complied. She volunteered that she had two girls of her own. She smelled good. Big brown eyes. Great smile.

I was witty and confident and I could tell that this random attractive woman in Walmart was into me. And I wished her a Merry freaking Christmas and walked away without getting her name or number. WTF?? I am not accustomed to having any game at all or any confidence when it comes to chatting up a strange attractive woman. At least not in a long time. This is new to me all over again. Shit.

I could beat myself up for the missed opportunity, but instead I'll take credit for at least flirting and talking. I can remember not so long ago when I would have said nary a word and been nervous just passing her in the aisle - scared to even make eye contact. So this is what progress looks like. Continuous improvement. And the next time an opportunity presents itself, I'll leave with a name and number or a polite no thank you. But I'll take my shot because my confidence is building each day.

12/25 Monday Day 75

It's Christmas! Today I am thankful to be alive and thankful for my family. And all the other blessings in my life.

Very little sleep from playing Santa, but overall I felt nice today. My mind and vision were clear and my mood was very solid. Peaceful. I realized at some point during the day that I did not have to consciously talk myself into a good mood even once. This is a huge change from the past million years of my life.

I pinned earlier today. And realized I was out of needles and only had some 31 gauge insulin needles. I am not even sure why I had them, but they were up in the cabinet so I attempted to use them. The HCG was no problem at all, although the short 5/16" needle seemed to leave a little ball of the fluid just below the skin. It felt like a little bead was under my skin so I massaged it until it dissolved.

But the testosterone. That was a damn circus trying to shoot it through such a small needle. First, it took like 5 minutes to draw the liquid up to my dosage level. Then it was full of bubbles. Then it would barely depress when I tried to inject it. Then I pressed too hard and it began to seep out of my skin at the injection site. So I pressed as slowly as I possibly could and eventually emptied the syringe, but the injection site began to burn badly. I rubbed it to try and massage the liquid into the muscle and it only burned worse. It freaked me out a little. I was worried I had some air bubble in the muscle that might go to my heart or brain and wreak havoc. But I was able to shake it off and go to the gym and put my focus elsewhere.

I felt fat and flat at the gym. My shoulders hurt. I weighed in at 187. I was uninspired. I watched a dude around 20 years old who I have seen lifting for the past 3 years rep out incline dumbbell presses like they were nothing and it pissed me off. When the kid first showed up in the gym he was soft and had small arms. Now he bulges in his clothes and has a killer physique. I always feel like I am starting over. I busted my ass for the last 7 years post-divorce, not counting the interruption from Lyme. And I have nothing much to show for it. I suppose that is one of the benefits I expect to get from TRT, but my ass better get motivated and dedicated if I expect to see changes. This is not a steroid dose. It is not magic. I still have to put in the work. I need to keep hammering that home to myself. Shit.

12/26 Tuesday Day 76
Man I feel great today. I had nice nocturnal wood and morning wood, even with a few glasses of whiskey last night to celebrate another successful Christmas. My mind was clear and focused when I awoke after 7.5 hours of sleep, and I felt ready to get shit done.

None of those big pimples either. My skin actually looks pretty good right now. I damn sure did not like those deep embedded pimples that just would not quite come to the surface to pop. Unsightly and aggravating as hell.

I took an Epsom salt bath last night after my workout, and I just lie there thinking about all the things I want to get done in 2018. Things I have been unable to accomplish in the past for various reasons. I had this quiet confidence that I can do it now. That it will take work, but I really can do it.

I'm talking about focused intentions on the 3 main areas of life: love, health, and wealth.

I finally beginning to feel confident enough that I can approach and flirt with most any woman. And I am learning enough to be able to get a date and escalate from there. Shit at 42 I should have long known how to do this, but somehow it just became apparent to me that I knew nothing about attracting and seducing women. How did I ever get laid in college? Beer I suppose. Lots of beer.

I have made a conscious choice to improve my health and enjoy life to the fullest. Lyme disease taught me that for sure. I only have so many years, and they go by quickly. So do whatever I can to look and feel my absolute best. Treat my body well with good food and challenging workouts and lots of rest and relaxation. And cut back on the damn drinking.

For the first time since maybe I was a naive kid, I believe I can be a millionaire. A truly financially independent man with an abundance of wealth and a magnet for money. At times I have dreamt of this - who hasn't? But now with a clear mind and a sense of real purpose, coupled with newfound confidence and a don't give a shit attitude about other people's opinion - I believe. I can see the path forward. I am unafraid of the work necessary to get there. I am ready to hustle. Finally.

I expect great things in 2018. I'll end 2017 with a crazy sex-filled weekend with Jewel to kick off next year in style. From there, any damn thing is possible.

12/27 Wednesday Day 77
Another excellent day. I woke up and did not hit the snooze. I said a quick prayer of thanks and then my feet hit the floor. Nice wood. Drank my coffee and began work immediately. Was productive for a couple of hours, then my ex remembered to tell me that Scarlett had basketball practice at 10 so I had to scramble to get her there. I just had this feeling of overall confidence while watching the girls practice. I even noticed at one point my posture was straighter. How'd that happen?

Today was the first day I took the pregnenolone/DHEA capsule I got from the compounding pharmacy. Not sure if it has had any effect after only one day, but at least nothing negative that I have noticed has happened. The dose is 100 mg pregnenolone/25 mg DHEA time released. Sounds good to me. I'll get bloods in about a month and see how it has changed.

My mind felt clear and sharp all day. We stopped by the market and Lexi was working. I chatted her up, then she chatted me up. I actually think she was responding to my confidence because in the past she barely stopped whatever she was doing to speak. Today it was like she could not get enough of me.

I worked the rest of the afternoon from home, then Scarlett and I hit the gym around 5. I felt more energy today. More focus. And I crushed a back workout. I took my notepad with me so I can start charting my workouts again. I found a decent Push/Pull/Legs routine on the web that I am going to run. It is similar to what I have been running with some different exercises that I don't often do. I need a change.

And wouldn't you know that as I was getting close to done Lexi walked in. Again she walked straight to me and smiled big and said hi. I do not usually get that response. Then a few minutes later as I was sitting at the curl machine, she stopped right in front of me with her ass in my face so I could get a good look. Tight black spandex with the outline of little panties that covered maybe 1/8 of her ass. And her ass is fine. Not bony or flat, but round and muscular. I cranked out a couple of extra reps just thinking about it. Then as I was leaving, she was hanging out at the front desk where I stopped to sign out. She mentioned wanting to do more cardio, so I invited her to run a 5k with me. Now it's on. I just have to find us a race and we are signing up. Shit was that easy! Who is this guy I am becoming?

But then tonight the bad news. Jewel called and said she has a kidney stone and can't come up this weekend. For some reason I had this feeling in my gut that she was going to cancel. No New Year's sex celebration. At least not with her. I suppose that opens up other opportunities. I feel like I'll be okay either way.

Tonight I am still working and writing and getting things done and I am honestly out of my comfort zone. But it is important to push myself and try new things, and do things that scare me. I just feel like getting shit done. I may even knock out another blog post. This is an amazing feeling.

12/28 Thursday Day 78

Woke up a bit fuzzier, but still feel overall great. I remember waking up at one point to pee with a MASSIVE erection. It was awesome. I just wanted to snuggle up with it and go back to sleep.

And when the alarm went off this morning I still had one. Good signs.

I do feel cold this morning. I think it is related to starting to diet again. It seems anytime I begin to restrict calories I get a bit cold. I am going to the gym to do abs and cardio soon and that will get my blood pumping.

As I was falling asleep last night, I woke myself because I had stopped breathing. Like something was caught in my throat. Time for the sleep study. I have always snored a decent amount, and I have read that TRT can make any apnea worse. I am taking no chances with it. Perhaps I can get by with a mouthpiece that repositions my jaw rather than full CPAP. I'll schedule it soon.

I pinned my testosterone this evening and it was perfect. I have the right size needles again so no issues. I have been alternating shoulders, but I think I'll do the quads some to avoid any scar tissue in my arms.

12/29 Friday Day 79

Felt pretty good this morning. I got up and went into the office and got some work done. I felt so extroverted walking around the plant which takes some getting used to. I just wanted to stop and chat with everyone, even the people who usually piss me off. I shook hands with the men and wished them a happy new year. It felt good. I felt alpha.

There was just a bit of brain fog that I noticed while sitting in the HR office discussing some things. Not bad, just enough to know it was there. This could very well be Lyme as opposed to anything hormone related. Or it could be a little of both.

I'm pretty stoked about seeing Kristi tomorrow night. Have I mentioned that? Jewel cancelled, and Kristi moved right into my life. How about that shit? So I'm excited. Not because I am interested in anything long term, but because I feel I can be outcome independent and just enjoy the evening. I won't be obsessing over what she thinks of me or whether she likes me or not. I will be there for my enjoyment, and I will look to offer some enjoyment as well. Either way I'll have a good time. And I might get to see some boobies.

I feel a bit bad for Jewel. She texted and said she had to have surgery to remove the kidney stone. She really was sick and not just blowing me off. Just shitty timing for both of us. I still intend to visit her soon and have a little fun.

I had a very nice leg workout this afternoon. I did not weigh in. The scale is deceiving me because even though I am only eating around 2000 calories a day and should be losing weight, I feel I am gaining muscle. My body composition is changing. My belly is beginning to lean out this week in spite of all the food I ate over the holidays, but my arms and shoulders and legs are fuller. So I will go by the mirror and how tight my pants are more than the scale. Maybe I am getting "newbie" gains even though I am not at a calorie surplus most days.

I feel really good about setting goals for 2018. In the past I have set goals and made resolutions, only to let them go and maybe only hit a few of them. But I have this inner confidence that I can get shit done now. So when I set goals it will feel like they are already pretty much accomplished. They will be realistic and attainable, and require good effort and focus and push me a bit out of my comfort zone. The way goals should be.

12/30 Saturday Day 79
Slept for 9 hours without moving and woke up with a massive boner. Perfect.

I feel like hitting the gym, but today is rest day. So I rest. Plus there are college bowl games on and I get to watch football all day and act like a man. Nice.

My mind is clear this morning. No real fog. And even though I am going out with Kristi tonight I am thinking about how I might pick up a girl between now and then for tomorrow night. It can be done. I am not sure the old me would have ever entertained such a thought.

12/31 Sunday Day 80
Woke up with great wood after sleeping for 8 hours. Mentally I was very alert and ready to get shit done. Man I'm looking forward to 2018.

My date with Kristi went okay. Not great, but it was okay. She looked much hotter than I was expecting when she walked in and threw me off whatever game I thought I might have had. We had a great conversation at dinner and I was making her laugh and getting her to open up, but I kept drawing a blank on how to move the situation past conversation. Like I just forgot that part of me that goes after the woman in front of him. I couldn't get comfortable and did not feel Alpha, whatever that feels like.

Things began to look up when we stopped by a liquor store on the way to a party and she bought a bottle of bourbon for us to share. I thought she might just get shitfaced drunk and things would get wild. But we both held ourselves in check and were just two nice people hanging out together. I did not feel studly in anyway and felt like I was getting friend zoned. At the end of the night I got a hug and a smack on the lips. And then she drove home.

The one positive I would note is when her lips touched mine I got an instant, massive boner! I mean the reaction time was like 1/8 of a second. If we had actually made out I might have burst through my pants! Which just made me realize that I could have been having crazy monkey sex with Jewel if not for the damn kidney stone.

Look at me. I have two hot women in my life where I had none before, and I am complaining about not having sex yet with either of them. 2018 is going to be awesome.

1/1 Monday Day 81
A brand new year and a brand new attitude. Everyone seemed to have the

flu or a cold last night, and it was 18 degrees in MS so no one wanted to do much. I ended up just hanging out with mom and dad and drinking dad's whiskey. It was a nice night with the parents. I'll be happy I had those when they are gone.

And I thought about what I want to get done in 2018. What I'd like to change. The man I want to become. I have never been more excited about a new year. I am about to start listing my goals for this year and man I am pumped. I feel like I can accomplish just about anything.

I have felt a bit bloated the past couple of days. And I had no wood this morning for the first time in a while. I wonder if estrogen has crept up on me. I am not scheduled to get blood work again for a month. Should I go ahead and request it be checked now? Maybe. I read on ExcelMale about some guys using DIM to control estrogen without having to use an AI. Maybe I will give that a try. I wish I had a daily estrogen monitor.

Hitting the gym at noon today. I expect to see lots of new faces in the next few weeks. Which means lots of new women. Am I ready? Maybe.

1/2 Tuesday Day 82
Woke up at 4 AM wide awake. My mind was buzzing and my body felt on edge. It sucked. But I think I know what caused it which will be a major breakthrough in my health if I am correct.

Before bed I took a big swig of apple cider vinegar and I noticed within 15 minutes my heart was racing. I was able to use deep breathing to get calmed down and drift off to sleep, but then woke again several hours later. I know when I was taking all the antibiotics for Lyme that my gut got pretty screwed up and I had candida. If that stuff is still hanging around then the vinegar would cause a large die off which would then cause a reaction in my body. Just like the one I experienced. So I am researching protocols to clean that shit up for good. There is plenty of research that demonstrates the connection between the gut and overall health. I am leaving nothing to chance.

On a positive note, I woke up later feeling much better with a nice stiffy to start my day. I felt confident and present and got a lot of work done before leaving for our hunting camp. I was even disappointed that I did not have time to stop by the drug store and get some Vitamin D before we left. I wanted to go in and flirt with Becky because I just feel on today. What a difference! I can recall going in there last year with my head down feeling so self-conscious that I would just murmur my words sometimes. Now I feel like I can talk to her with my head up and actually have something interesting to say. Progress!

1/3 Wednesday Day 83
I only slept about 5 hours. I woke up with a buzzing in my brain at 3 AM. Really feel crappy today. And I am convinced my hair is thinning. I have not had it cut in well over a month. Usually in that time frame it gets thick and unmanageable. But it is thin and dry. It has gotten longer I'll admit, but it is just not as thick. And my hairline has moved maybe half an inch in a month. Hopefully this is as far as it goes. I posted a question about it on the Testosterone FB page, and I only got two responses. Both suggested DHT was the culprit but neither suggested any solutions.

I can tell my libido is shit right now even though I am not having sex. The last time I went hunting, I sat in the stand basically fantasizing about sex the entire time. Now it seems I could care less. I even wonder why I was so excited about my date with Kristi or getting to see Jewel. Shit.

1/4 Thursday Day 84
I slept better but I was so damn tired from the night before it would have been impossible not to. I woke up to go hunting again at 4:30 AM and had a damn raging boner. But still don't feel all too interested in sex or anything else right now. It's time to get my blood done to check on estrogen I know, but my work schedule is not cooperating right now. I might could squeeze in a trip when I get back tomorrow. We'll see.

I keep getting these damn big pimples on my chest. Like 3 or 4 at a time. 2 will fade then 2 more will pop up. It's pretty aggravating. I'd be self-conscious about them if I had a woman around. I'll keep using my Proactive body wash and hope it gets better. I wonder if there is something else to use.

My mood is flat but stable tonight. I was too damn tired to go to the gym when I got back from deer camp. And I am bloated from drinking too much while there. I am going to really try and limit alcohol for the next little while. That is sometimes a challenge when there is not shit to do in the winter, but it is damn difficult to lose much body fat while drinking nearly every day.

Some of that New Year's motivation is already waning, but I am determined to make this an excellent year so I will keep myself motivated one way or another.

I wonder if I need an AI if my estrogen turns out to be high, or if I can use some other supplement or diet change. If I did have to take one I am sure it would be low dose. My estrogen was always too low before. Like really low. I doubt I suddenly became a high converter, but who the hell knows? Pretty frustrated tonight. I keep looking for a change in my life and just when it seems things are getting better I get knocked on my ass back to where I was. My mindset has changed, but the circumstances seem to always stay the same. Surely with a change in attitude comes a change in reality. How long does it take? Shit.

1/5 Friday Day 85
Slept hard last night, but woke up feeling clear and ready to go. It's so damn cold out right now that the bed felt awesome this morning and I could have stayed there all day. But I have shit to do.

I have looked for evidence of hair loss and can find none. Even though my hair feels thinner and my scalp is itchy, there is no hair on my pillow or in my shower drain. I suppose I could get a new hair brush and monitor how much comes out in it, but maybe I am just obsessing. I do need a trip to the salon because the back is shaggy and uneven so at least it is growing some.

My mind has been on point and I have been 100% productive for over 3 hours now at work. I can say with certainty that this was not the case in the past, even before I got sick. My mind would easily wander and I'd get distracted and lunch time would arrive and I would mostly have shit to show for it. Now I am productive and efficient - or at least I am today.

1/6 Saturday Day 86
I feel very bloated and fat. My belly was hanging out yesterday like I have been putting away a 12 pack daily for months. The truth is I have had maybe 6 beers in the last month. Whiskey is a different story, but it's not like I've been drinking it by the gallon.

This morning my face looks full as well. Very moon-facish. I awoke with no morning wood and in fact everything was kind of drawn up and lifeless. Now I do recall getting up to pee around 2 AM and having such a monstrous erection that I had to sit down on the toilet to avoid spraying the walls. That was nice. And kind of freaky. Maybe it was a dream.

My mood is somber and that feeling of confidence and wanting to get shit done has faded again. Is it the passing excitement of a new year or is it hormones? I need labs to tell the full story, but I feel unmotivated to make it a priority. It seems to just come and go at will, with no rhyme or reason. Perhaps I should monitor the moon phases. Makes as much sense as anything else in my life.

Scarlett's first basketball game was this morning. I noticed while sitting there that there were no thoughts running through my head. At first I was worried that I was zoned out or that my mind was broken, but then I thought maybe I am just not over thinking and obsessing about everything. Then I zoned out.

I did feel kind of strong which was weird. I ran into a guy who beat me up in grade school. He is still a head taller than me, but I felt like I could take him for some reason. And I kind of wanted to. That was a strange thought to have at 42 years old.

And my ex-wife was there with her hubby. At first they sat down on the other end of the gym, but when the people in front of me moved they moved down and plopped into those seats. My ex was hanging all over her Neanderthal husband right in front of me. Now I am not jealous in the least. God bless this man for enduring this woman. But it still pissed me off a bit that she was making such a display. It pricked my ego enough to want to go out and find the hottest blonde I could and parade her at the next game. But that won't happen because these games are about my daughter. So maybe I'll find a hot blonde and parade her somewhere else. Either way it let me know that I can still be motivated regardless of what is going on with my hormones. Damn right I can.

1/7 Sunday Day 87

191 freaking pounds! That is what I weighed at the gym yesterday evening. I knew I felt bloated, but damn I have not weighed that much since I was fat and married 7 years ago. I am beginning to seriously doubt that TRT is doing anything but making shit worse.

And Lexi was there looking hot as hell in black spandex pants, and I was too ashamed to even look at her due to my moon face and flabby gut and lack of confidence and absent libido. Damnit man.

Scarlett and I went to the movies last night and watched Jumanji. It was funny, and I realized I was totally zoned out while watching it. Not thinking of anything else except where we were which was nice. But I believe it had more to do with a good dose of brain fog than anything related to a healthy psychological state.

There was a cute blonde in front of us with no ring who looked to be in her early 30's. Someone I might have struck up a conversation with only a few weeks ago. Last night I was just hoping she wouldn't look my way and give me a look of disapproval. Shit. If this is all simply estrogen related I suppose I'll laugh about it but man it sucks. I had to drag my ass out of the recliner to even go to the movies. I could have easily fallen asleep and chilled all evening. After getting over 8 hours sleep the night before. Low energy, low libido, low focus, low motivation. I had all of those before TRT and I did not even have to stab myself with needles.

But at least I woke up with a raging erection for no one to enjoy but me. It looked huge next to my tight scrotum. Shit.

1/8 Monday Day 88

I woke up at 4:47 AM wide awake. It wasn't so bad. I was expecting it because I took a big dose of ACV before I went to sleep. It just confirms what I suspected about candida. Somehow I forgot to go online and search for home remedies for this, but it will be priority today. Something to do while I travel to Toronto. It's 4 damn degrees there with a 90% chance of snow this evening. Awesome.

I pinned my HCG last night. My stomach skin must be getting tougher because the last few pins have hurt like hell. Like the needle has trouble penetrating, then it suddenly pops in sending a bolt of pain through the tender area. Maybe I should consider smaller needles for the HCG. The 27 gauge seems just right for the test, and it rarely hurts the tougher area on my shoulders and quads. I'll discuss it at the clinic when I go back next month.

I will not have time to get labs this morning before I leave for the airport. It will have to wait until I get back. I suppose one more week at this point won't be too painful. I considered skipping a dose to see if I feel better, but that would mean my labs would not represent my current dosage so I'll just keep on.

Emotionally and mentally I cannot really complain. True there is some brain fog, but there is no depression or anxiety and I feel fairly positive. Maybe a bit frustrated but certainly not down and out. I just keep telling myself I'm almost there and a spectacular fucking day is just around the corner.

My chest acne seems to have settled down. The Proactiv wash has helped, and it has mostly faded now.

7:02 PM Well, my anxiety kicked in about the time I boarded the plane from Memphis to Detroit. I thought I was going to have to come off that fucker. It felt like a gorilla had me in a bear hug and thousands of needles were pricking me everywhere. I was able to deep breathe my way through it and settle down a bit once we were in the air, but damnit man it sucked. I really, really hope this can be attributed to high estrogen. If I get that shit checked and it is spot on along with good testosterone numbers, then I'll be left scratching my head as to what to do. This could end up being the point where I jump off the TRT wagon and just endure as best I can and hope that my natural T can be optimized enough for a decent life. What a freaking let down that will be after having such high hopes of everything getting better. But it is what it is man.

1/9 Tuesday Day 89
My self-discipline is severely lacking. After settling down from the flight, once I got to my hotel I hit the bar instead of the gym. Like I was programmed and could not deviate. I had 4 beers and some chicken nachos. Not my finest moment.

My sleep was kind of shitty, and I woke up with no wood in a sour mood. Serves me right I suppose. I looked doughy and just beat in the hotel mirror. Perhaps I am.

The day has been kind of spacey but semi-productive. I did feel some depression creeping in but I did my best to ignore it. I really do not like that shit at all.

My libido is non-existent. I am in downtown Toronto with hot girls walking up and down every sidewalk. I have reading some things online about conversation openers and feel I know enough to at least strike up a conversation with an attractive woman. But right now I could care less. If one offered to show me her tits I'd tell her it's too cold and put them away before she gets ill. Tricky fucker, that libido.

And honestly, all the pickup and seduction shit does not work if you don't really believe it. If you cannot see it happening and think there is a chance, than short of ponying up the cash to hire a coach that will force you to do it, you are likely to stay stuck where you are. Maybe if a person could spend some time working on their inner game before going out into the world and attempting outer game, they might have a chance. But everything I have read is approach, approach, approach.

3 MONTHS IN

1/10 Wednesday Day 90
The 3 month mark. Progress is mixed so far.

My sleep last night was restless. It seemed anxiety was just flowing through me. That was after a nice gym session, a healthy dinner, no booze, and meditating. I sure hope it's just high estrogen.

I woke up feeling buzzed with a semi-softy. Better than nothing. Overall I felt pretty numb though.

Yesterday I began a gut cleanse. No grains, sugar, or alcohol. Up the healthy fats, eat some fermented foods, and lots of ACV. I found a fermented cayenne honey drink at a Canadian pharmacy by the hotel. Sugar free. It was actually quite tasty. And I had a bowl of greens with chicken and avocado from a health store across the street. So far so good. I did feel less bloated this morning, so that's promising. But this damn anxiety has got to go. The depression too.

Brain fog has been elevated today. At lunch with colleagues I had trouble following the conversation. And on the drive back I almost forgot I was in Toronto on business as I stared blankly at the factories and warehouses we passed. Fun stuff.

And I keep feeling hot and flushed. My face and brain feel full - like hot water is flowing forcefully through all the veins and cavities in my head. Weird.

1/11 Thursday Day 91
I slept better last night. A solid 7 hours I would say. And when I awoke I could have driven nails. I just lie there admiring it for a few minutes before arising for my day.

And I look leaner today. A few days of low carb has at least drained some of the bloat. Still looking forward to knowing my lab values so I can make adjustments if necessary. And I get a haircut tomorrow. I wonder if my stylist will notice anything different about my hair. It's actually pretty shaggy right now, so I was incorrect in thinking it is not growing. Receding a bit maybe, but definitely still growing. And not as itchy as it was.

The large chest pimples are gone, but now there is kind of a rash of small ones. 10-15 of the suckers. Very unattractive. But none on my back where I used to see them. Weird. Of course I am using hotel soap and not my Proactiv, so perhaps that is contributing. I have some zit cream but my skin is already so dry from the winter weather I really don't want to use it.

The boys are not hanging very well this morning, but can't say it's much of a priority right now. I really just want to feel good. Little details like that are not enough to worry about. They are still there, so I should just be thankful. Shit.

1/12 Friday Day 92
I slept great last night. 7 solid hours without even getting up to pee. I was wiped out from Toronto.

Woke up in a much more positive mood - like a fog had been lifted. I pinned last night around 11 PM when I got in from the airport. Both test and HCG. No problem with either injection.

Today I was supposed to get labs, but we had a damn freak snow storm in Mississippi and Scarlett got to stay home from school. A few more days won't hurt. I am positively getting it done Monday morning.

Had a strong leg day in the gym this evening. Even did squats again with some decent weight. I had been avoiding them since my hernia operation, but I used great form and did not push too hard. My legs felt nice and rubbery afterward. And I weighed in at 186. Down 4 lbs. from last week. So I lost a lot of the bloat.

I am seriously considering a cycle while on TRT. Once I get a little more time in and get more comfortable with managing labs/dose/sides, I see no reason not to. Lyme disease taught me a lot, and some of the main things are:

Life is short so live it up
Don't take shit too seriously
If you want something, go get it
Have some damn fun
Don't give a shit what others think

There is plenty of info on the forums for how to accomplish this. The big thing is having extra testosterone. I have maybe half a bottle from my botched run on TRT while deathly ill from Lyme. I don't think that is enough though. Perhaps if I let my levels fall down some before I go back to the clinic he might prescribe a higher dose. Or maybe I can order some off the internet. I don't know. It's just something I'm thinking about doing. Especially if I lean down like I want. Why not build some serious muscle? I am 42 years old. I spent two years in hell from illness. My confidence with women was sucked away by low libido and ED. I want to reverse all that and have some damn fun for a while.

My mood has been pretty freaking awesome all day, and I got great shit done working from home. This is how I wanted to feel. Not all bloated and anxious and depressed like I was only a couple of days ago. Amazing how quickly things can change. Still lacking libido though. Can I judge libido without a woman around? Likely not. So I'm really making too much of that aspect and just talking myself into not having libido. Perhaps if I got off my ass and went and found a woman, then I could gauge libido. If only there was a book on inner game...

1/13 Saturday Day 93
Today has been pretty decent, although I woke up with no wood for the first time in a while. Just soft. And definitely still no libido best I can tell. In fact the thought of sex is quite foreign to me right now.

I took my daughter to the mall and we had a nice time. I was foggy though. No depression or anxiety, but I was kind of floating along. I did notice several attractive women smile at me as I passed by, but I honestly just didn't care. Maybe that's the secret. Not caring. I have that covered for sure.

Not only was there no wood this morning, I have been drawn up tight all day. And not just my boys. Mr. Wiggly has also been drawn up like he was trying to get back inside. It's been hell taking a piss without getting any on my hands. It is cold out, but it seems more than that. Why can't I be normal? I remember being normal at one time.

And even though I have had no anxiety today, last night as I was drifting off to sleep I had an acute feeling of someone grabbing my throat and clamping down. I sat up in bed and it felt like electricity buzzing through and I struggled to catch a breath. Freaked me the fuck out. But I was able to cough forcefully and break the spell, then I settled back down and did some deep breathing to get relaxed again. I was able to sleep a good 8 hours after that. Weird. No scratch that. Not weird. Just my fucking life.

1/14 Sunday Day 94
I slept very well last night, but no wood this morning and Mr. Wiggly is hiding again. If Lexi from the gym showed up and offered herself I would have to send her to the neighbor's house because I couldn't do shit with it.

I had a low buzz of anxiety when I first woke up, but I did some deep breathing and it released. My mind is semi-fuzzy but functional, so that is what I am working with today.

My chest is pretty broken out today. It sucks and looks pretty bad. My biceps seem bigger though. And my gut is beginning to go down just slightly. Perhaps if I had an estrogen spike it has resolved itself on its own. Today is HCG pin today, and I am finally getting labs done tomorrow.

Also, if my hair was beginning to recede or thin, it has since halted. It seems okay right now and feels pretty normal again. Maybe it was just really dry from the dry winter air and seemed like it was thinning. I hope so. I have damn nice hair.

1/15 Monday Day 95

No wood today. Everything soft and drawn up. I feel less bloated though and my face appears thinner in the mirror. That is much more pleasant to look at. I had no confidence at all with moon face.

My mind is quite clear this morning, and my mood is very positive. Perhaps the most positive it has been in a couple of years. The derealization that set in with Lyme seems to have lifted a bit more in the past few days and I feel like a better version of myself. I don't know how else to describe it. I will never feel the way I did before getting sick. It just changed me too much from the inside out. But today I at least feel real and part of this world and grounded. The only thing at all to even remotely complain about would be the drawn up state of my goodies. Maybe that is about to be resolved as well. I am so ready to start dating again.

I drove from Mississippi to Ohio today. Took about 10 hours, and not once in that time did I have even one anxious breath. I take no anxiety meds now. No benzos. No SSRI's. Just vitamins and good old testosterone. Shit. It was a nice and pleasant drive and I had overall blissful feelings when observing the countryside from the Interstate.

Better days have found me.

1/16 Tuesday Day 96

I had weird sleep last night. After driving for 10 hours, I had this slight buzz in my head of nervous energy. I wanted to go running instead of go to sleep. But at midnight I forced myself to relax since I knew I had a full today of work. I slept 7 hours and woke up less fuzzy than most days. No wood at all. Drawn up and kind of puny. But I felt good!

Today at work I have been uber productive. I can recall so many days spent in this Ohio cubicle wasting the day away instead of working. I just could not focus very well before, even before I got sick. Now I am tearing into stuff that I would have easily avoided in the past, and it feels damn good.

I get this sex thing resolved, and I could be a man on fire.

1/17 Wednesday Day 97

I only got about 5 hours sleep, but I am not sleepy. I napped last night after I got to the hotel. I had actually laid down to meditate, but ended up drifting off for about an hour. So I got up and went to the hotel gym and then ate dinner.

After that I worked in the room until midnight. I was just so focused and intent on being productive. Where has that been the last 40 years??

I finally drifted off around 1:11 AM. When I woke up I had no wood, but my mind and mood were pleasant. Then I got half wood while just lying there thinking about the day ahead. My boys were still drawn up though, and now feeling kind of soft.

I have been productive again today at work. I took time to book two trips to New Orleans over the next few months. One is a work conference, and the other is a concert. I am confident in my ability to find companionship for both, in spite of my lack of dating life at the moment. Shit is about to change.

I called the Wellness Center to get my lab results but no one answered. Perhaps they were gone to lunch.

Something interesting happened at lunch today. I ate at this little cafe here in BFE, Ohio. When I went to pay my bill, there was a cute country look-ing girl working the register. I said nothing to her, and as I left it dawned on me that not so long ago I would have talked to her and flirted a bit. I had that little feeling of an edge briefly, and now it is gone. And I want it back.

This afternoon I have had restless energy, and my face feels warm and flushed. Hot flash? Maybe. I am focused but still kind of floating, if that makes sense. I know for certain the depression and derealization are not present. That is a blessing. But I still want more.

1/18 Day 98

No wood at all this morning. I woke up in a foul mood but shook it off.

It started last night at dinner. I was eating with an old friend of mine, and mid-conversation my mind fogged over and I felt stoned. I shook it off, but when I got to the hotel instead of being productive I just lie in bed and read random shit on Reddit until I got sleepy. I did sleep okay but woke up disappointed and wondering if change is truly possible.

The shower seemed to wash the blues away and my mood improved some, but I was all drawn up still and it just pissed me off. I feel like my fucking life is on hold until I get this sorted out. Low libido. Low confidence. Complete performance anxiety. Wanting to date and enjoy what's left of my youth, and watching painfully as the days tick away. Fuck.

I hoped TRT would be a step in the right direction. That it would bring me out of the pit that was Lyme disease and depression and anxiety and help me enter my best chapter yet. And maybe I've seen glimpses of that, but I am still sleeping alone and still celibate not by choice. This shit has got to change. Soon.

1/19 Friday Day 99
Almost 100 days in. Over 100 days with no sex. This is bullshit. But as my buddy says, "it is what it is".

I slept about 5.5 hours last night and woke up with plenty of energy and in a solid mood. Maybe a little anxious but not terrible. But no wood and very drawn up. So tired of that experience. How the hell can a man develop confidence with that going on?

And wouldn't you know it, but after finally getting my ass to the clinic for labs they get a snowstorm and are closed all freaking weak. So it will be Monday before I find out if I need an AI or if something else is going on.

Brain fog is definitely up. I catch myself zoning out and struggling to call up words. I was trying to think of those hard things that make up the shape of my face earlier and couldn't quite place my finger on it. Then it hit me - bones. My face is made of fucking bones.

1/20 Saturday Day 100
Rough morning. We woke up early to deer hunt, and I really wanted to lie

in bed. My brain was buzzing and my breath was a bit ragged. Anxiety pretty damn high I'd say. It's hard to get comfortable when this shit is going on. I worked through it the best I could.

I had a chance to take a nap this afternoon and passed. I wanted to have fun with the men from deer camp and hang out and shoot the shit instead of being by myself. That is definitely a change from how I used to be. But still, this damn anxiety has me just feeling out of sorts. And zero libido. Can't even stand the thought of pussy right now.

My mind is wandering back into some of the obsessive thoughts like it used to do. I'd compare it to being in mental wrestling match with some dark entity that seeks my total destruction. Very uncool shit.

I noticed earlier my chest acne is worse. And I have these large pimples on the back of my head and some on my neck. These damn things are deep, and very painful. Shit.

1/21 Sunday Day 101

My mind was total fog this morning. I drank too much last night and slept fitfully. It felt like someone was clamping down on my throat while lying in bed. I hate anxiety.

Still, even though my mood tried to be sour I kept talking myself into a better place. I just liked it a hell of a lot better when that good place came natural. When it was my set point instead of somewhere I strived to get to.

I really, really want to see those damn labs. I just feel uneasy as hell in my body right now. This is not panic or extreme anxiety, just an uncomfortable feeling that leads to fear that leads to self-loathing that leads to wondering how much I can take. It's a vicious cycle that I end up having to consciously break. Where is all the good shit in my life?

This evening at the gym I did a half-ass chest workout. The impingement in my shoulders is so bad that pressing just about anything is a no-go. I focused on slow cable crosses and dips and anything else that did not pinch, which wasn't much. I'll do some research on shoulder exercises for impingement. Probably some stretches or some shit to magically fix it.

I felt a little better after the workout though. Like I was able to channel a bit of the anxiety into the movements and release it.

Scarlett and I had a nice healthy dinner and watched some TV, and now it's time for bed.

1/22 Monday Day 102
I slept nicely for about 7 hours. No wood at all when I awoke, but I did not have to get up once to pee which is nice. It wasn't so long ago that I was waking up 4-5 times a night to pee when my hormones were extremely low. I remember when my estrogen got down to single digits, I could not retain any water and my joints popped like bubble wrap. At least my balls were full back then though.

I had the low buzz of anxiety when I first woke up, but I meditated and it eased up just a bit. The clinic opens in 20 minutes so I'll have my answer soon enough. One thing I have avoided thinking about is what to do if my numbers are good. Check thyroid again maybe? Cortisol? I know I cannot accept this feeling. It is not sustainable and makes no sense when I got to a point of ZERO anxiety not so long ago. And I think I was having nice erections but now it's just a memory. I can go back and read through my journal and see I suppose. It was an excellent idea to track this. Hell, I might even share this journal with others online if it would help them. I probably would have read this if something like it existed.

3:28 PM Just heard from the lab. Estrogen was high just as I expected. It was 62, up from 28 back in December. My other numbers were high also. Total was 1200, and free was 37. No results yet on DHT. Not sure why the total number have gone up so much. I'm still using 100mg per week. At 186 lbs. I think that is about right. Perhaps the labs were at close to peak levels according to my metabolism. I can't imagine that being a trough level. I'll take .5 mg Arimidex twice per week and retest in 30 days. Hopefully I feel better. Strike that. I <u>will</u> feel better.

1/23 Tuesday Day 103

I slept well last night. About 6.5 hours of solid sleep. I awoke with a nice stiff one, then dozed for a few minutes and when I woke up again it was gone. Progress. The low buzz of anxiety was not there this morning. I'm not sure if the .5 mg of Arimidex I took yesterday afternoon can work that fast, or perhaps the 5k I ran at the gym yesterday released some tension. Or maybe just a placebo effect. Whatever the case it was not there today.

Brain fog is a bit better, but it was already getting better before I took the pill.

I posted a question on Nelson's Facebook Page asking how long it typically takes for Arimidex to kick in. I got some helpful responses, with one guy saying 24 hours and some others a bit longer. Then there was the usual "tell me your protocol" posts that people throw up there no matter the topic. It's like they are convinced their dosage/injection frequency is king and they cannot wait to critique yours and tell you how wrong you are. I ignored those. If I had specifically asked for input it would be different, but come on. I've read enough to know that 100 mg/week broken up to every 3.5 days, with 250 mL of HCG taken also every 3.5 days is pretty damn standard. I could tinker with it some, but I am not one of those yahoos who come on their taking 200 mg every two weeks wondering why they feel bad. Next time someone asks for my protocol, I'm asking for theirs so I can tear it apart. No, that would be a dick thing to do. I am not a dick. I think I still have one despite its lack of use, but I myself am not a dick.

Today I have been productive but not necessarily highly motivated. I also realize I cannot rely on TRT to properly motivate me. That comes from within. It just has the potential to reduce roadblocks.

Yesterday I read online where the gentleman who created Peaktestosterone.com was killed in a car wreck. That's so damn sad. I learned so much from the site over the past few years. That dude genuinely helped thousands of people to improve their lives.

It puts things in perspective a little bit. Most of us are on a quest to be the best version of ourselves. To answer a calling to be more than we have been. And even if we are able to rise up and answer that call, there is no guarantee it won't all be taken away tomorrow.

So let go of my damn fears and live, damnit!

1/24 Wednesday Day 104

I crushed my workout last night at the gym. I had a pump like I used to get back in high school and college - maybe better. A weird thing happened while I was there. A friend of mine, who happens to be cute and married, stopped to say hello. I have hung out with this girl and her husband many times. I have been drunk with them and always enjoy carrying on with both of them. But for some reason there was this awkwardness between us. When I said hi and asked how she was doing, she got all quiet and shy around me. It was weird as hell. I don't know what to make of it. Part of me wants to believe she was suddenly attracted to me and did not know how to react, but the other part of me thinks maybe she sense something wrong with me or thought I was hitting on her or something and just did not want to be around me. Hard to say.

There were a couple of other cute girls in there, but none of them paid me much attention. I focused on my workout and kept my mind in a positive place.

I have made the shift to a lower fat diet from my traditional high fat high protein diet. I feel good so far. Maybe that helped with the pump having all that glycogen from extra carbs. This week I have been eating oats, rice, chicken, tuna, salad, protein powder, sauerkraut, and Greek yogurt. I think that is about it. Been shitting a lot which is good and gives me time to catch up on world events.

I woke up in a good mood with no anxiety this morning. I had decent wood but not great. Boys were drawn up. I have been intermittent fasting which makes me cold. Could that contribute to the drawing up of the goods? Maybe.

Around 9 I left work and went to the local clinic to get a lipid profile, thyroid profile, and ESR checked. I am curious as to what my inflammation level is compared to when I had Lyme. It gotten high as a giraffe's ass when I was really sick. My ex-wife said she didn't know CRP could get that high. I am hoping inflammation is no longer an issue.

The cute redhead who usually draws my blood was not there. I had sly intentions of getting her number if the opportunity presented itself. Instead I ended up in an awkward silence with hot brunette at the front desk. I say she has a pouty face. My ex-wife says the girl has resting bitch face. She is cute enough and at one time I thought I might ask her out. I totally choked on that opportunity a few weeks ago at Walmart, and now whatever momentum I thought I had there has passed. She rarely smiles, has 3 kids, been divorced for only a year, and has small tits. So I am telling myself those are the reasons I don't go for it. Feels better than calling myself chickenshit in front of the mirror.

Anyway, I'll get some lipid numbers to see how I stand and what adjustments I may need to make. Always good to know.

Mentally I am in a good place today. I feel very relaxed and content. I do notice a lack of drive, but give me a day or two to adjust not crawling out of my skin and I'll get my groove back.

1/25 Thursday Day 105
Like a gypsy wandering the desert, I trudge on across the sands of no sex hell.

My sleep was weird last night. As I fell asleep I felt like I was being pulled down into a pit. I woke up feeling okay. Pretty damn good actually. But by noon I wanted a nap. Time to get a sleep study I think. I just have this inner knowing that I am not breathing deeply during sleep.

I woke up with no wood today. It was disappointing since I thought after taking .5mg of Arimidex I would see a big difference. Not yet I guess.

It was a productive work day, and after work I took Scarlett and our dog to the golf course and we ran sprints while he chased us. It was awesome. Then we went to basketball practice and I just had this overall feeling of wellbeing sitting there watching. It was awesome too. She went with her mom afterward, and I came home and finished a blog entry I started a week ago. I edited it and added graphics and posted it and added it to my FB page. It was not difficult at all. I love that damn blog and when I get more people reading it I think it will really help people. Posting more than once per week would easily drive some traffic. Right now I am at about once per month.

I got my labs back today. ESR was 5 which is good. Thyroid looked good. TSH = 1.68, FT3 = 3.4, FT4 = .72 which is a little low but not bad. My cholesterol was not so good though. Total was 199. Not terrible. But HDL was 35 and LDL was 164. That ratio must change. I took my first Red Yeast Rice pill tonight. I'll check again in 60 days to see the effects of that plus my Mediterranean style diet. No fucking statins for me, buddy.

I think more cardio can also help. I ran a 5k Monday, and I ran a mile yesterday for time. I was going to do legs tonight, but I've been at the gym 4 nights in a row. I'm going to write some on my Lyme novel then take an Epsom salt bath. Hopefully the warm water will thaw out my drawn up balls.

1/26 Friday Day 106
I slept great last night. I woke up just before the alarm was set to go off, and had decent wood. My boys felt a bit fuller this morning. The best part was mentally I just had a feeling of wellbeing that has not been there in a really long time. Like everything was just super-duper. It has been here all day and made the day so very damn nice.

My bed was so comfy and cozy I almost slept in, then I got up and thought I'd just work from home. I thought if I went to the plant everyone would see me coming in late and pick at me about it. Then I realized I gave zero fucks what people there think of me and I went to the plant.

I was very productive until noon, then came home and took a nap in the recliner for about 15 minutes. I love that I can do that right now in my job.

Although I feel better overall, my confidence is still not where I want it to be. I still hesitate a lot instead of moving forward or just going for it. I still over think a lot of things, which is a lifelong habit that will take some time to let go. But I do feel better. I like that.

Even with some hesitation, I have this deep inner drive to succeed. To prove to no one but myself that I can do this thing called life. That I can be the best version of me and focus on health, wealth, and love. That I can live without anxiety and let life flow for me. I know it will never be perfect, but damn it is not meant to always be a mountain to climb either.

It's a Friday night and I have nothing to do. My social life is not where I want it to be any more than my romantic life is. Even my best old buddy from high school was in town with his wife and had a cook out at his new house. They didn't invite me. WTF?

I can recall before I got sick with Lyme, that it seemed like someone was always texting about something going on. Once I could no longer participate, those people just faded away. I bear them no ill will. Everyone has their own life to live. If I want a better social life, then it is up to me to get one. Let the weather get a little better and I'll have a nice cook out of my own.

The idea to have a wine and whiskey tasting at my house has crossed my mind several times. I've even discussed with a few others and had good feedback. Will I follow through? In the past that would be a big no. We'll see.

Sometimes I have these thoughts of being a social hub in our little boring town. Of hosting routine cookouts and themed get togethers. This town is so damn sad sometimes, but it doesn't have to be. It was fun growing up here. It can be fun again.

1/27 Saturday Day 107
I woke up nice and firm and clear this morning. Just right.

Last night I wrote on my blog and in my Lyme novel. I cleaned up around the house. I had a great leg workout at the gym. I drove to Corinth to try and pick up chicks at the Walmart (did I just fucking type that?). And I took a nice long soak in an Epsom bath before bed. Only one thing missing and there is no need to mention it. But soon maybe.

I picked Scarlett up for her basketball game, then afterwards she and I watched TV while it rained outside. We had dinner this evening with the whole famdamily, and it was fun! I jabbered on and on which is a complete 180 from how I usually am around my family. It was like all the little things that normally piss me off about them were suddenly gone. My mom even asked about my job. I'm 42 years old and I think it is the first time she has ever asked about what I do for a living. It was like living a dream. Damn I had a good time.

1/28 Sunday Day 108
We overslept just a bit and missed Sunday school. I slept for 9 solid hours and it was amazing. And I woke up stiff and happy. Good things are here!

After church, Scarlett went with her mother so I came home and meditated. I considered going to the gym, but I was a little sore from Friday so I went hiking instead. I took the dog and we hiked for about 2.5 hours up and down some pretty tough hills. But it was glorious. I basked in my good mood and debated if I had ever felt so overall blissful. It was a little scary at times because that feeling is so new to me. The AI was just what I needed. If I get much better I'm not sure what kind of life I'll be living! I was hoping so much to run into an attractive woman. I just felt "on" and knew I could flirt and carry on like a ladies' man if given the chance. But it was just a bunch of dudes and one couple. Still, the hike was awesome. It worked the stiffness out of my legs and gave me a nice opportunity to reflect on the hell of the last couple of years. And think about what I want in my life now.

There is a lot of uncertainty, but two things are clear:

I want to feel good.
And I want to help people.
Everything else is just icing on the cake.
When I got home I felt so productive that I did laundry and knocked out another blog post. That's two in one weekend! I used to struggle for two in one month.
Yep. 2018 is shaping up to be the best yet. I love it.

1/29 Monday January 29 Day 109
Well shit. After feeling so great all weekend, I began to feel some anxiety last night as I got in bed. I felt kind of flushed throughout my body and just did not feel comfortable. I pinned my HCG yesterday earlier in the day without issue. Except I must have hit a vessel in my belly fat because it shot blood when I withdrew the needle. First time that has happened with my stomach. But that would not explain the anxiety.

And after hiking all afternoon, getting shit done on the computer in the evening, and taking a nice Epsom salt soak, I should have been completely relaxed, right? I even had a glass of red wine before bed. So why the anxiety? Did a week of AI result in my estrogen going too far the other way? Did I pass my sweet spot only to now be too low? Damnit man!

This morning I pinned my T, but I did not take my AI. I am thinking I will take only 1/4 pill when I go home for lunch. Perhaps since I was only around 60, taking a full 1mg in a week was just way too much. I noticed my wood was kind of hard but skinny this morning, and I peed a lot yesterday without really drinking a lot of fluids. Just like I used to when I was sick and had low everything. So the roller coaster continues.

10:24 PM I'm about to go to bed. The day got better as it went on. I took 1/4 AI at noon, and I worked productively until 4. I picked up Scarlett and got suddenly sleepy on the way home. But I resisted a nap and instead worked on the Bronco with her help. We pulled the rear axle out of the rear end because it has a leaking seal. It was pretty cool and she enjoyed helping her dad.

After that it was basketball practice, and even though I had some brain fog, I was in a better mood and the anxiety had subsided. Scarlett went with her mom afterwards and I came home. I almost succumbed to sleep, but manned up and hit the gym. I ended up completing a very nice push workout. I am definitely getting stronger. It's a damn shame my shoulders have impingement. Otherwise I am quite sure I'd be setting PRs on bench right now. But I am content to work around the pain and use dumbbells and cables and machines. My chest is shaping up nicely and I have pecs again for the first time since college.

My mind has also been very creative tonight, and I had a brilliant idea for a 30 day course on becoming a better dad for your daughter. I know nothing about sons so it would be specific to raising girls. First I will try it out, then I will share it. Maybe it will help someone.

There was an attractive woman there but I did not get her name. There was just never a good opportunity to talk to her, or at least I told myself that.

1/30 Tuesday Day 110
I woke up with great wood this morning and in a great mood. The anxiety that showed up the other day is now gone. I honestly think it was more related to gut issues. I had taken a large amount of ACV Sunday night, and I have seen in the past that it can cause a reaction when the yeast dies. I should have known.

My mood today has been one of getting shit done and just feeling like good things are happening even if I can't see them yet. I worked 8 hours, picked up my daughter, ran a couple of miles at the gym, ate dinner with my mom, and now I am watching Donald Trump give perhaps the most strategic SOTU address I have ever seen. I watched most of GWB's and a few of Obama's. They were very polarizing with one side standing and clapping while the other groaned. But the Donald has outsmarted them again by speaking to things that no one can sit and groan on. Families of children murdered by MS-13. Money for infrastructure that includes government and private industry. Tax cuts for all. A 12 year old boy who started a movement to put flags on the graves of veterans. And then I spoke to soon. He just rolled out his 4 point immigration policy, and no Democrats are clapping. Oh well. It's still better than most.

I have good ideas and creativity flowing again. I feel like good things are on the way. I feel good physically. If anything just a touch of brain fog but nothing like before. My mood is so much better and positive. The chest acne is clearing up since I began taking the AI. Just a couple of bumps now. If my hair receded at all, it has stopped. And damned if my chest and belly aren't a bit hairier now. I was wondering if I would see those changes.

1/31 Wednesday Day 111
This week is dragging by for some reason. The days just seem long. I awoke with decent wood, but I long for those mornings where I had wood that was so engorged I thought it might blow the head off. Am I being greedy?

I was a little bit sore. One thing I had noticed is that my muscles have not been as sore after working out these past couple of months. But now they are getting sore again. When my testosterone was low, they were always sore unless I stayed completely out of the gym. Even before Lyme. But recently not so much. Perhaps it is just a matter of getting T/E ratio right. I would like another draw after starting the AI, but I suppose I should give it a few weeks and then check it. If I check it all the time and constantly adjust, I'll never have a chance to settle out. So onward we go.

2/1 Thursday Day 112
I awoke with nice wood this morning, but my sleep was not so great. I woke up with that inner buzzing sometime in the middle of the night. I did some relaxation techniques to go back to sleep. Not sure why my sleep is inconsistent. Still need a sleep study. And some sex.

Yesterday after work I did feel a bit of anxiety, but I chose to ignore it and just kept on doing what I was doing and it just disappeared. Maybe after all these years of anxiety it is just a challenge for the body and mind to let go of it completely. Maybe. Either way I felt good and had a nice back and biceps workout. Very nice.

I was a bit disappointed to discover the kid I have worked out with for a few years who is just out of high school is on gear. I had thought he was just making exceptional progress over the past few months, but he had on a tank top last night and looked like he has gained 30 lbs. or so of solid muscle. And his back and shoulders were covered with acne and huge pimples. He couldn't just be satisfied with a great physique at a young age. I suppose I should mind my business. I just hope he has someone guiding him to do it right. Hell, who I am I to judge? I am contemplating running a cycle at 42 myself. I am definitely adding some muscle, but the belly fat is slow to come off and the muscle gain is slow as I am mostly eating at maintenance calories for fear of gaining anymore fat. Either cut or bulk man, make a damn decision.

As for my boys, apparently they are on a damn yoyo of some sort. Up and down, up and down. They have a mind of their own, so I am paying them no mind at all anymore. If I knew how to fix it I already would have, so just let it go.

2/2 Friday Day 113
I woke up at 5 AM feeling great. I could have driven nails, my mood was positive, and my mind was clear. I visualized, meditated, prayed, and got up to write. I think this is how all mornings should begin for me.

Last night instead of lifting, I ran a 5k at the gym. 33:34 was my time. I got a stitch in my right side around 1.5 miles so I had to stop and walk for a bit. My goal is to run a 5k in under 30 minutes, which I know I can do.

I pinned effortlessly last night. I am so proficient now. I can do it in under a minute while Scarlett is in the other room. I still have not told a single person I am taking this therapy. I guess it's just personal.

2/3 Saturday Day 114
I'm in Gulf Shores to paint the condo this weekend. The drive down yesterday was very nice. I felt positive and strong, although I was bloated again and did not like the puffiness in my face. I have eaten clean all week, no booze, lifted and ran, and I'm puffed up like a marshmallow. Whatever.

I still slept soundly and have been painting steadily all day. It's nice being able to enjoy visiting the beach again. I've had some damn horrific trips these past couple of years where I came here to relax but felt so bad I just watched in misery as the waves rolled in. Now things are better.

Mom and dad are down here helping me paint. I used to get so damn pissed when dad offered any amount of criticism, but now I feel so centered and confident in who I am I just shrug it off. He means well.

We had dinner at Sea n Suds and there were attractive nice looking ladies serving. I only got one of them to smile at me though. Oh well. The entire restaurant was full of geriatric snowbirds. The servers were probably tired of getting hit on by men who reminded them of their grandfather.

2/4 Sunday Day 115
Superbowl Sunday! I've got $200 on the Pats. Can Brady do it one more time?

I fell asleep around 11 and slept soundly until 6:15 AM. I awoke with zero wood and was a little disappointed. I meditated and fell back asleep, and when I woke up at 8 I had wood. So I guess I just got a head start on Mr. Wiggly and had to let him wake up.

I'm not as bloated today. Must be the beer I drank last night working as a diuretic. Either way I feel lean and muscular today and look good in my painting t shirt.

I was observing how good the condo looks now painted bright blue, and thinking ahead to when I might spend some time here with a woman. I have not had a woman down for a beach trip since around the year 2000. What year is it now?

We have finished painting and have been debating on getting some seafood to bring back here and watch the game. But I feel like being out and around people, so I suggested we watch the game at Acme Oyster House. You never know who might show up.

2/5 Monday Day 116

I woke up before daylight with a mess to clean up. Apparently I had a wet dream. At 42 years old. Weird. I guess at least I am getting some action in my sleep. Ha ha.

After that I went back to sleep and awoke again around 8 AM with a weak morning erection. Whatever sweet spot I have it is a challenge staying there. Is it worth the trouble? So far it's a wash, even with the improved mood.

I noticed after my shower this morning that the chest acne is back. That's just awesome. A few days away from home and my Proactiv body wash and I look like a leper. Bumps on my back too. I guess it's time to start travelling with the body wash.

My mind is clear this morning though. I do like that. And my mood is somber but positive. I did lose $200 on the Pats last night, so that has a little to do with my mood not being any higher. But Brady can only do so much. A defense giving up 41 points and a million passing yards is too much to overcome, even for the GOAT. Maybe next year.

BEGINNING TO SEE THE LIGHT

2/6 Tuesday Day 117
Good wood, good mood! The day started off right with me sleeping 7 hard hours and waking up ready to go. No grogginess, no wanting to snooze. Just eyes wide open and ready to drive nails.

I worked with such focus and concentration it was sometime after lunch before I realized I was hardly speaking to anyone. I got a lot of shit done today.

We had a group company dinner and I felt relaxed and sociable, and I did not feel the urge to drink anything at all! I was the only one at a table of 12 people and it did not bother me one bit. I talked and laughed as much as anyone, and got to watch a few coworkers get a little bit sloppy and unprofessional as the drinks kept coming. How many times has that been me?

I did eat way too much though. For some reason I was hungry and ate appetizers, salad, entree, and dessert. I rarely eat that much, and now my belly is swollen and ugly. Not a pretty site at all. Especially with chest acne to go with it. I had a big painful pimple right in the middle of my chest when I got back to the hotel room. Damn these torturous invaders!

There was a table of very hot ladies around 30 years old beside us. While a couple of the guys were ogling them knowing they would never have the courage to talk to them, I was thinking of what I might say to them. I am starting to feel some confidence - but what to do with it? Take the plunge and make a move.

2/7 Wednesday Day 118
Damn life is good today. I slept a solid 7.5 hours. I mean I did not move except maybe I peed once. It could have been a dream. I did not wake with any wood, but before I went to sleep I got the hardest damn erection I've had in years. I mean I had to feel of it to make sure it was real. The damn thing was like solid steel.

I will note that since I was travelling and skipped my HCG earlier in the week that my boys were drawn up considerable after only a few days. Would I trade that piece of steel for some drawn up nuts? I would think so. But I am positive it is not a tradeoff. Just a matter of adjusting.

But my mood. Man I just want to get shit done. Be productive. Suck up the abundance of life. Dance naked in the street. Howl at the fucking moon. Maybe whip somebody's ass if they get out of line. Who am I becoming?

2/8 Thursday Day 119
I woke up with raging wood. Had to sit to pee to avoid spraying the wall. I'm a little puffy from eating too much this on my work trip this week and not working out, but my mind is clear and sharp.

It's difficult right now to relate to what it was like before. Being locked up in my head, full of anxiety and self-doubt. I have not even had sex again yet I am confident in my ability to do so. It's hard to explain.

My shoulders are hurting even though I have not worked out this week. That kind of sucks. I need to be more consistent with my stretches.

Work was a breeze today. I debated working from home, but I wanted to be around people. Did I just write that? I wanted to be around my coworkers and get shit done and help where needed. And I did. I even stayed until 5 PM though it was not necessary.

I picked up my daughter and we went to Walmart, where I ran into Miss Resting Bitch Face again. This time there was no awkwardness. I smiled and said hello and accused her of following me. She smiled and laughed and made a funny comment. And that was it. I left it on a high note. Now the next time I see her we will have something to laugh about, and she will have a positive memory of me to draw from. This shit isn't so hard.

And something else interesting happened. I ran into a different girl I know, and after just saying hello and mentioning I was looking for Scarlett since we had gotten separated, she dropped what she was doing and led me around the store to hunt for my daughter. All the while she chatted me up, and then when we found Scarlett I could not rid of the girl. She talked and talked and looked me up and down several times. I think she would have mounted me right there in the store. Now this girl is crazy and not suitable for dating by any means. The words "don't stick your dick in crazy" were first uttered in reference to girls like her. But I also acknowledge that a night in the sack could be pretty fucking wild with her. I could not initiate such an event with my daughter there, but I am certain I made a down payment on something if I can work it out discreetly. Hey, even I have a reputation to uphold.

We went to basketball practice and I felt tuned in and comfortable. My ex from junior high was there and even though she has added a few pounds, she is still pretty. I had this odd urge to just tell her how pretty she still is. I could barely stop myself. But she is married now so I was able to refrain from possibly making her uncomfortable.

And that was about it. We came home and I had a light dinner of oatmeal and almond milk with protein powder, and we just finished watching Shark Boy and Lava Girl. What a great movie! It was about bringing your dreams into reality which really hit home with me and is a great message for kids. And the best line of the movie: "Selfish dreams don't deserve to come true". So whatever I'm planning for the future, make sure it's not just about me.

2/9 Friday Day 120.
Another great start. I woke at 6:15 AM ready to chop down a tree, then I meditated and got up and made coffee.

After getting Scarlett off to school, I commended myself for not getting frustrated at her for not being completely ready by 7:40 AM. My calm, clear mind allowed me to shift focus on everything she did right: make the bed, get dressed, put food and water out for her dog, brush her hair, get her books together. The only things she missed were fixing her drink thermos and brushing her teeth. In the past I would have pissed and moaned about those two things and we would have parted in foul moods. Not today.

Even though my diet was shit this week, I am not really any fatter. It's like I have a higher tolerance for imperfection right now. I will say that my eyebrows continue to fade. They are but whisps now. Is that something to be worried about or just a trivial observation? Shit, I just don't know.

I drove to Tupelo because I thought I had an appointment with my therapist, but it is not until next Friday so I just chilled at the mall for a bit. I got a coffee at Barnes & Noble and read a book on making small talk. I searched for an attractive woman but only saw a college aged girl doing homework. Would I have approached an attractive woman if she had been there without a ring on? I'm anxious to find out.

After that I stopped by PetSmart and did end up having a wonderful 10 minute conversation with a complete stranger on how we treat our pets like babies. She was a married black woman about my age, and I started chatting her up while selecting dog food. Next thing I knew she is showing me pictures of her family's dog on her phone and giving me her life story. I have struggled for decades to connect with people, and now I am making friends with married black women at the damn pet store. Who am I becoming?

2/10 Saturday Day 121
Another good night of sleep. I could get used to this. Nothing special in the wood department this morning. Is the old saying true, "If you don't use it, you lose it?" Surely that can't be so. Perhaps I should become a monk.

My legs are a bit shaky today after a killer leg workout last night. I mean I pushed it. I had such a pump in my quads it was to the point of being uncomfortable. I have not had such a leg pump since college I'm sure. I almost threw up a couple of times.

My neighbor's son was there. He must be close to 25 now. Been on the juice probably since high school. He's totally inked up and a monster. His chest and shoulders are just massive granite. I wonder if it's worth it. He seemed happy enough. We spoke for a moment and he mentioned that he was home after serving a few years as a marine. Somehow he maintained his size during his service, so I'm guessing he had access and Uncle Sam does not test for such things.

This evening we had the Daddy Daughter dance. My little girl looked so beautiful. I teared up in the picture line when a dad and his little girl were standing in front of us. She looked to be about 3 and he was just holding her in his arms while she rested her head on his shoulder. Both of them perfectly content with the world. Oh I wish I could have captured those days with my daughter and just relive them anytime I choose. I am fortunate that I recognized how fleeting they were at the time and enjoyed every second. I knew better than to waste them and have to look back on the missed time spent with my daughter. I spent mine wisely. We have gone everywhere together and done everything together since she came crying into this world. And still it's not enough to satisfy my desire to keep her my baby forever. Would I have more kids at my age just to enjoy those loving moments again? Perhaps.

As I sit here thinking about my plight with women, I acknowledge that it is not all driven by carnal desire. It is driven more by an intellectual knowing that experience with the opposite sex is healthy. Perhaps when up close and personal with a woman that carnal desire would be unleashed, but it is not present at the moment regardless of how long it's been since I have had sex.

2/11 Sunday Day 122
No wood this morning. I was tired at church and in a somber mood even after a decent night of sleep.

Not a bad mood. Just somber. I felt frustrated a bit and felt like nothing is happening in my life right now. No women. No social life. No new opportunities. Just work, spend time with daughter, exercise, and spend time around here wondering if life is passing me by. I blame it on living in a small town of about 3000 people, but the truth is I'm just not creating my own opportunities right now. At least I don't want to eat a bullet. My mood is positive most days and I am thankful for it.

So many things are good. I don't feel so much like hanging myself or walking out into the ocean in the middle of the night. My skin is not crawling with anxiety and my vision is no longer distorted like I'm tripping on acid. No joint pain. No paranoia. I'm mostly positive with a general knowing that life is pretty good. But I want more damnit.

I hit the gym this afternoon. That was after my 2 hour post church nap. There were a handful of people in there, but no attractive single women. If I lived in a large city where the gym was full of hot women, would I take my shot and go after some of them? I like to think so. It's easy to just go to our little gym day after day and recognize that it's the same married gals trying to lose their baby fat. This is my comfort zone. I long to break free from this. I could drive 25 minutes to the neighboring town to work out and have many more opportunities. Something to consider.

I'm eating too much. I've gained some nice muscle, but my damn belly is nowhere close to flat and my face is nice and round. Even when intermittent fasting I am eating too much. My appetite is just more than it used to be, but my daily caloric needs have not increased that much. Something's got to give.

2/12 Monday Day 123
Another great night of sleep. 8 solid hours. I woke up in a much better mood with positive expectation for the day. And had nice wood to greet me. Does consistency ever come?

I worked for 4 hours from home and was very productive, then drove to the pharmacy 35 miles away to pick up more testosterone and AI. I also got a refill on the pregnenolone/DHEA compounded capsules while I was there. I wonder if that stuff just aromatizes, and if I quit taking it could I quit taking the AI. Something to consider. It's hard to say if there are any positive results from taking the supplements. Maybe I'll post it on Gene's FB page and see what the bros say. I already know what they'll say. "What's your protocol bruh? You should be doing x,y,&z."

This afternoon I ran about 4 miles at the gym which felt great. I had to walk part of it due to shin splints. I'm not sure if it is the shoes or the treadmill which causes those. I never got them much before Lyme when I ran outdoors all the time. I suppose I could run outdoors and discover the answer pretty quickly. Maybe the weather will be nice this weekend. Maybe coyotes will chase me down and eat me alive.

I weighed 187 at the gym. Not bad considering I've eaten a lot the last few weeks. I'd still like to lose this gut. Strike that. I am losing this gut.

That's about it for today. Lexi was at the gym but I did not get to speak to her. She was huffing away on the stair stepper when I got there, and she left before I finished running. Maybe tomorrow. And her ass looked awesome.

2/13 Tuesday Day 124
Interesting day. I woke up well enough. Another good night sleep but not much wood to speak of when I got up.

I pinned yesterday around noon. It's supposed to be Monday AM, so I am making a note to stick to my schedule better.

For the past couple of weeks I have backed off of the iodine I was taking in the form of Lugol's solution. I thought maybe those high doses were not healthy. The result is I've been freezing cold at times, with poor circulation in my hands and feet. My fingers were like ice last this evening. After Lyme disease, will I ever be right again?

And not to be outdone by changing my iodine dosage, I also elected to up my AI to .5 mg this morning instead of .25mg like I had been taking. I thought maybe since my libido and drive weren't so great it could be that estrogen is still high. Plus I have the residual body acne that is just being stubborn. I know labs would be nice, but damn I can't run to the clinic every couple of weeks. I was supposed to take 1mg per week anyway, so it's not like I'm taking too high of a dose.

By the end of the evening I felt anxious. Even a little shaky. So is it the

AI or the reduced iodine? I checked my body temperature and at 7 PM at night it was 97.4. I don't think that is acceptable. Maybe I'll see a naturopathic doctor in the same town as my wellness clinic and check levels of lots of different things and discuss how to optimize thyroid if that is what is lagging. What a damn seesaw. My awesome life.

2/14 Wednesday Day 125

Last night was weird. I was shaky and cold when I got in bed, and even though I was tired I was also a bit wired. Seeing my low body temp coupled with having a stiff neck gave me flashbacks to the hell that was Lyme. I started worrying about low thyroid and crashing estrogen and all kinds of other shit. I drifted off to sleep only to wake up gasping for air in a near panic attack. It shook me pretty good, but after Lyme that kind of shit is not too scary. It used to be a nightly routine. I was able to slow my breathing and relax and drift back off to sleep. I wonder if the AI was too much. Can it even work that quickly or was I just stressed seeing the low body temp? Hard to say.

I feel better at work today and am not so cold. I put two drops of Lugol's in my morning water so maybe that shit helps. Who the hell knows at this point?

2/15 Thursday Day 126

My sleep was fitful last night. I was tired but wired again. I could not relax even with a guided meditation, which usually knocks me right out. I finally drifted off then woke up at 4:30 AM wide awake. I dozed until about 6:30 then got up.

I did get decent wood around the time I woke up, and my mood was better than yesterday. While in the shower any brain fog I had seemed to lift completely for a moment, and I felt pretty good all morning.

My intentions were too fast all day until 7 this evening, but I was weak and ate a FIT crunch bar when I went home for lunch. And a Quest bar. Oh well. My will power could use some work.

Since I took the .5mg of Arimidex, I have peed like crazy just like I used to. I read something about low estrogen making it difficult to retain fluids. And I feel leaner like I lost a bunch of water. I wish I knew what it was now. I pin again this evening and am unsure if I should take anymore. Maybe just a .25mg dose. I am my own science experiment.

My pull workout last night was intense and I found myself pushing for extra reps where I would have stopped a few months ago. My back felt flushed when I got done and my arms were pumped. And not too sore today. The DOMS I routinely experienced before is only very mild now, with the exception of shin splints which I did not get before.

I ordered a candida cleanse for my gut last night. I am excited to see what it can do. No telling what kind of yeast I have after all the Lyme meds I took. The reviews from people who had struggled with gut issues about life-changing experiences were motivational to say the least. People talking about decades old symptoms resolving themselves, dead yeast coming out in their shit and piss, and all kinds of other super powers. Fun stuff! I should take some pics and put them on FB if my shit glows in the dark.

2/16 Friday Day 127
I was a bit foggy this morning. Not bad, but enough to aggravate me. Not much wood either. I want to wake up and conquer the world. I want to crush my enemies. See them driven before me and hear the lamentations of their women. Who said that?

Most of the day I was just kind of in a daze. My mood was positive and I definitely enjoyed just being alive which is nice, but I felt no particular motivation or drive to do much. I just wanted to relax and chill. I'll take it.

This evening I had a killer leg workout again. I am really enjoying those and seeing some size on my quads for the first time in a long time. I weighed 185 which means I dropped a few pounds of water weight by giving up grains for Lent. Why do I eat grains at all?

I opted to not take an AI this week. If I begin to feel bloated and moody and foggy again I'll take that as a sign that my estrogen is creeping back up, but I think it got a little too low based on my joints and skinny erections. We'll see. The wild ride continues.

2/17 Saturday Day 128

It's been a great day but I am beat. I woke up feeling good and in a positive mood with nice wood. I attended my daughter's basketball game this morning and felt very alive and in the moment. I was outgoing and talkative and just felt in the flow.

Afterwards dad and I worked on the Bronco all afternoon until dinner time. I felt very manly working on an old 4x4 and getting grease all over me. After a couple of bowls of chili for dinner and some red wine, we watched Narcos then I came home. I soaked for an hour in an Epsom salt bath and felt so good when I got out. Then I realized I was alone again on a Saturday night. I would take some action if I knew what to take. But what the hell do I do? There are like 5 single women in this town that I might consider dating, and all of them bring baggage and potential conflicts of some sort. There are no bars or nightclubs to go and try to meet people, and my gym is full of married women and teenagers. I don't want to just give up and use my small town as an excuse, but damnit man! Enough is fucking enough.

It's time to give internet dating a try. I dabbled in the past and got one date with a girl who turned out to be not so attractive in person, but it did not matter anyway as I was just beginning to get sick and everything got put on hold.

Jewel has found someone. Kristi doesn't seem too interested and I'm not either truth be told. Plus she is 70 miles away. What's left? Keep spending my Saturday night's alone watching TV with my dad? Shit. I guess I should be thankful my dad is still around and I am not suffering. But still I want more.

2/18 Sunday Day 129

After the great bath last night, I slept like a damn rock. I mean for 9 hours or so and almost missed church. Apparently in my haste to fall asleep I never set the alarm. But I made it. And I had a big fat erection when I got up.

My body looked leaner in the bathroom mirror, but I have some puffiness in my face. Could be the red wine I drank last night.

But my mood today has just been out of sight. The candida cleanse pills are already helping as my mood has been more stable and more of the brain fog has lifted. I am onto something with this stuff. The gut is a key part of health. Who knew?

Looking back at when I was sick, it seemed the really bad brain fog set in after I was taking doxycycline for a while trying to get rid of the Lyme infection. I always assumed it was the infection itself causing the fog and mood swings, and maybe it was to a point. But the damage to my gut compounded that and apparently extended the suffering longer than needed. I'll continue to make an assessment as needed.

I also felt more motivated today. I spent the day hanging out with my daughter, but I felt more motivated to really start getting things done again. To take massive action in all parts of my life and see what happens.

Working on the Bronco yesterday with my dad was a good lesson. He has always been a man of action, but it did not transfer very well to me. I've lived a life of leisure in many regards, always dreaming of the future and putting things off. A lot like a young Luke Skywalker. My dad just gets shit done. I probably would not have worked so diligently on the Bronco without his urging. But he kept after me and once we were committed we were both all in. And we got a lot done along with some good father-son time. There was no anger like there might have been in my younger days. I'm too centered and present for that now. And he has certainly mellowed as he has gotten older. He's still teaching me if I'll just pay attention. When something needs to get done, just fucking do it.

2/19 Monday Day 130
My sleep was pure shit last night. I was full of energy at 10PM and could

have gone to the gym right then and crushed it, but I wanted a good night's sleep since I am driving to Chicago today for work. I had trouble drifting off, then I could not stay asleep. I just had the electric buzzing throughout my body that prevented any relaxation. Not really racing thoughts. It was physical more than mental. I must have slept some though because I had some good dreams about a couple of women who have passed through my life before. They were not sexual in nature, but perhaps some meaning as one of them kissed my cheek with loving eyes and the other properly ignored me while I properly ignored her. Or they were just random ass dreams about women I rarely, if ever, see.

I'm about to pin then load up for Chicago. Since I'm driving it will be easy to pack my pins for Wednesday and Thursday. Overall I feel pretty damn good considering my lack of sleep. And I felt leaner again this morning despite eating a healthy amount of calories yesterday. This Mediterranean style eating with no grains is pretty effective so far. I look forward to better lipid numbers at next check. I look forward to lots of shit these days.

I also had a vision on breaking my dry spell with women. Since I have been lazily using my boring ass small town as an excuse for zero opportunity, I had a thought smack me in the head of where to meet women without a cheesy online dating account. Start signing up for races in the area. Not only would I have the opportunity to meet nice women, but they would be either in shape or committed to getting in shape like me. There is one pretty much every damn weekend within 60 miles of here, so get off my ass and find them. And run baby. Just run.

2/20 Tuesday Day 131
Sleep was much improved last night. I drifted off a little after 10, and woke up once to pee then right back to sleep until about 6:30. I feel calm, clear, positive, and focused today. I am thankful for this day.

My morning wood was odd. It was hard as steel but not engorged at all. Skinny is a good word. I took .25mg of AI yesterday with my pin, but no way it worked that quickly. Maybe just an odd penis thing. My penis can certainly be odd.

The drive up to Chicago was pretty cool and I felt so relaxed. Zero anxiety, even when I got into traffic and pouring down rain. I was just cool as a cucumber.

I flirted a bit at dinner with my Swiss server, and although she did not seem too interested I certainly felt outcome independent. That is a big step for me. I just enjoyed the interaction.

I can also tell that my urination frequency has gone back down. I know when I took the full .5mg that I shed some water and started peeing all the time the way I used to, but now I can drink a lot of water before I have to go. Just another observation.

Overall I have been productive today and my mind is sharp can clear. I look forward to a productive afternoon and a good workout. I wonder what my blood pressure is.

2/21 Wednesday Day 132
My sleep was pretty lean last night. I was on the computer past 11 which never helps, but even before then I just felt wired when I should have felt tired. I lie there trying to relax into a meditation and just had trouble getting my mind and body to let go. At some point I drifted off and got maybe 5 hours of sleep. And the weird thing is I am not sleepy today. Could it be that I just need less sleep now? I was sure enjoying getting 8-9 hours a night, but if I am okay with 5-6 perhaps I can adjust my routine and gain some productivity out of this instead of lying there lamenting my lack of sleep. Just a thought.

Jewel texted me last night. Things did not work out with her new guy, and now she wants me to meet her in Gulf Shores for a little beach romp. I know I should have more options by now, but I am learning to let go of my shoulds and just go with it. So first chance I get I'll be romping at the beach. I certainly have the tools to do some drilling now.

The past few days I've been a bit bloated in the gut and face and it was aggravating, but this morning it seems to be discharging. I have already peed 4 times and it's only 10 AM. I have had no water and 1 cup of coffee. This is good though. Ole moon face is not a good look for someone with already chubby cheeks.

Everything else is still good. My mood is positive, my outlook is optimistic, my focus is singular and effective. I am thankful and determined and in a good place. And I know this is how good things come to me.

2/22 Thursday Day 133
Barely slept at all. What is going on here? I worked out at the hotel, met a couple of colleagues for dinner, went back and read and watched a little YouTube, then turned off the lights at 10 PM. And I just felt wired. Nothing was really bothering me or running through my mind. My body just seemed to not be producing any melatonin or whatever triggers the sleep cycle. I had so much energy I could have just gone back to work. Or to the gym.

I put on a sleep meditation and was able to drift off after an hour or so, only to wake suddenly at 12:45 AM ready to go. I mean wide ass awake. So I just lie there for I don't know how long and drifted in and out until the alarm went off at 5:30 AM. And I felt fine. Not sleepy at all. I realize I may need less sleep, but I am positive I need some sleep. I'm not a damn vampire.

What is different about this week? I have not been taking my Lugol's iodine. I started taking the gut cleanse. I've had red wine most nights with dinner. I took .25mg of Arimidex after skipping a week. That's about it. I guess that's a lot, actually. I have not been consistent with the AI at all, and I know that stopping Lugol's can cause immediate effects like cold extremities. So when I get home I'll start the Lugol's back and stay consistent for a couple of weeks at least, and take .25mg of AI twice a week until my next blood draw which is coming up. And save the wine for the weekends. No need to drink it every night. It's good for the heart, but that is not a license to be a lush. I had great sleep only a week ago, it cannot be too far away from where I am now.

I will add that my balls have absolutely been hanging low since I started eating breakfast again. Fasting just makes me cold and draws them up for whatever reason. I like them hanging.

2/23 Friday Day 134
Slept pretty well last night. I woke up a couple of times but was able to drift back off. Much better than the previous two nights. The drive home today was peaceful and I got all excited listening to some YouTube videos on overcoming fears and becoming a new person.

My gym session this evening was short and intense. I hit legs pretty good then got the hell out of there. My knees may need wraps when I squat now. They just don't feel too stable even with lighter weight. Something to consider. Getting old ain't for pussies.

I pinned when I got home after lunch. So I'm about 16 hours behind schedule. Not too big of a deal I guess, but I should have taken a pin with me. Need to stay consistent.

Overall my mood has been excellent and my mind clear. Just looking for opportunities.

2/24 Saturday Day 135
I slept about 8.5 hours last night. I got up twice to pee, and each pee was a long one. Not sure where all the fluid came from. Balls nice and full this morning. I'm certainly enjoying having them back.

My daughter had her last basketball game and I felt so good during it. Just had an air of confidence about me and felt "on". Afterwards we went to a birthday party for my cousin's 3 year old and I was just yacking it up with everyone and playing basketball with all the kids. Not brooding in the corner like I have for 3 decades or so. It was cool! I believe my relatives think I'm on drugs.

Not much else going on. I have felt good all day and could have gone for a run but just ran out of time. I was down to 183 yesterday at the gym and my pants are definitely a little looser. 175 I think is a number where I start to really look cut. Especially with the added chest, arm, and shoulder muscle. I know it would be even better if not for these damn sore shoulders. It is paramount that I find a good shoulder rebuild program and stick to it.

My legs are not even sore today after hitting them yesterday. That used to never be the case. And it was 80 degrees today - the first day for shorts this year. My calves had some decent definition to them - just snow white!

Another good day is complete. I look forward to a good night's sleep.

2/25 Sunday Day 136

Another good night's sleep. Great wood. My days are becoming repetitive. These entries will only hit the highlights and any changes going forward.

I will say this about church. Pamela sat beside me today. The cute young blonde I pined over a few years ago when she was single but I felt she was out of my league. I mostly stammered gibberish when she would sit by me then. Interview type questions with no confidence or emotion. I felt pretty pathetic when around her. She invited me to play tennis with her one time and instead of immediately confirming a date I nodded and grinned like a drunk possum, no clue what to do with such an invitation or what it might mean. I wanted her but was terrified of her. She lives in Memphis and eventually her trips home have become fewer and fewer, until I only see her once every few months. At some point last year I discovered she had found a new boyfriend. It must be a tall, handsome, muscular rich guy right? Nope. A guy who looks about my age except he is fat and a complete ginger. I guy I would laugh at if you told me he had a shot with Pamela. I did not understand at the time.

Fast Forward to today. They are still dating. She is moving out of Memphis to the suburbs of Hernando, MS to be closer to him and their tennis buddies, and I felt like a total alpha male talking to her this morning. I greeted her with a huge smile and immediately drew her into my world. We talked more this morning in 10 minutes before church than the last 5 years combined. It was ethereal to some degree. She could have talked to me for hours. I wasn't just lusting after her and picturing what was under those tight dresses she wears to church. I was engaging Pamela the woman. I was showing her Rowdy the man. If she were single I would have gotten a date right then and there. After the service she continued chatting me up until she had to walk a different direction, smiling the whole time. She was probably wondering where the hell the new Rowdy came from. I wonder the same myself sometimes.

2/26 Monday Day 137

I slept from 10:30 PM until 4:30 AM, then I was wide awake and ready to get shit done. I mean I had to settle myself down because I was so ready to go do something. Anything. But what the hell do you do at that time of morning? I ended up visualizing and meditating, then I got up and cleaned up the kitchen and made breakfast for me and Scarlett. We were ready and out the door just past 7 which was perfect. No rush. No fuss. Just a nice sweet morning with my daughter.

I flew to Montreal today. I think my body wanted to generate some anxiety, but the best I could do was some butterflies in my stomach. It was a nice, mostly uneventful flight. I definitely have some altitude apnea though. On the leg from Detroit to Montreal, I drifted off several times and stopped breathing. When I would wake up it would take me a moment to get my breathing back to normal. It was pretty scary but I've had worse in the past. Not a good idea to sleep on the plane I guess. I wonder if there is anything short of a CPAP you can do for that. If I ever take a long flight someday I'll want to sleep.

My days are pretty redundant right now. Good sleep. Good mood. Drive to do stuff. Positive internal dialogue. I know it's just a matter of time before things change on the outside, but damn this wait! Still plenty to be thankful for.

I will say my boys pulled a disappearing act today. Not sure what is up with that. I am sure they'll be back tomorrow. Nothing else to write about to-night except I thought I looked better in the hotel gym mirror. Just a look of health I have not always had. That's a good thing I think.

2/27 Tuesday Day 138

I woke up in a foul ass mood. I slept well enough. Around 6 hours and then wide awake. But damn I felt like the weight of the world was on my shoulders and there was no point in getting out of bed and going to work. Like no matter what I do shit never changes. It was a damn shitty feeling.

But I was able to shake it off and get going and by the time I got to work here in Montreal I felt pretty good. Since then I have been productive and focused and in a neutral if not positive mood. Sometimes I think about the fact that I am 42 and how much time I have wasted over the years. Particularly these past few years both before I got sick and after. Getting divorced put me so out of whack and was compounded by living in a small podunk town with no one else to go out with. Then I got sick and a few more years slipped by, and now here I am putting shit back together before I turn 43 and hoping for some good years before old age catches me.

On the way up to wonderful Canada I was thinking about vacation options for me and Scarlett this year and the thought of surfing lessons crossed my mind. At first it was a nice image, but then the thought of maybe I'm too old to learn to surf crossed my mind. It is the first time I have ever thought I might be too old to physically do something and it just made me sick. And then I thought about how I have always wanted to write and how I've stopped and started over the years and just never got shit done. So maybe all this shit is surfacing as I count the days where nothing seems to be changing or happening and I just feel like time is slipping away.

All I know to do is keep working each day towards something better. Look to continually improve myself and take advantage of opportunities, and be prepared to create opportunities where none currently exist. What the hell else will I do?

One very positive note is that while I did not have wood when I first awoke, it showed up while I was preparing to enter the shower and I could have hammered nails with it. Like I was 15 again. Just need something to hammer.

2/28 Wednesday Day 139

Very productive day. I just seem to get shit done these days. I could have retired years ago if I was always this effective!

I have felt good, slept pretty okay, noticed my boys are drawn up again, and maybe a bit bloated. Do I need more AI? Only labs can tell for sure. When do I go back?

Last night I had dinner at a rooftop bar and restaurant overlooking Montreal. I thought about how I would have been full of anxiety eating somewhere like that before with glass walls hundreds of feet in the air with nothing but wide open spaces around me. But not now. And the cute French Canadian bartender seemed to like my Mississippi accent. I was very flirty and got her talking and laughing a little bit. Some guys would have just ogled her then went home and masturbated. But not me. Onward!

3/1 Thursday Day 140

Another new month. Shit this is going by fast. I slept okay last night. Had a glass of wine at dinner and wrote about 2000 words in my novel with my laptop at the hotel restaurant. Most work I've done on it yet. It felt good to feel like I accomplished something at the end of the day.

I had a raging boner this morning when I got in the shower. Just like old times! I have skipped breakfast this week but my boys are hanging in there.

Mentally I was in a good place. No anxiety for any of my flights, even when my plane got stranded on the runway due to a freak snowstorm. It snowed so hard you could only see a few feet across the tarmac. They tried de-icing the wings but they iced right back up, the flight was cancelled and now I'm in a shitty airport hotel room digesting a shitty steak from the hotel restaurant. Life is good.

I should have gotten home early afternoon and pinned this evening. Now I am off schedule again. Might as well plan on travelling with my injection kit from now on instead of trying to make it home in time to pin.

My weight loss, after making a bit of progress, seems to have stalled again. I know part of it is me travelling and drinking wine at night. But I'm still exercising and not eating over 2500 calories. And I like wine and a little bit is good for the heart. Guess I need to keep it under 2000 to move the scale. I can do that. I will do that. And less wine. But I do love it!

3/2 Friday Day 141
I woke up feeling nice and rested in spite of the shitty day at the airport and shitty hotel. Wood was a little disappointing and I felt kind of soft and bloated. I would like to be making better progress considering I am in the gym 3-4 times per week. Maybe it is time to change up the routine and push myself a bit more.

The flight home was smooth and I was so comfortable. Not a bit of anxiety, just like I like it. I was calm and focused and even began listening to an audio book to learn Spanish I have on my phone. My company is purchasing plants in South America, and if I want to be a key player I need Spanish. Having the focus and determination to learn a new language at 42 is pretty cool.

This evening after I picked up Scarlett we had dinner with the family. I was in such a good mood and felt strong and outgoing. Not locked up in my thoughts the way I was for decades. My family is getting to see a better side of me.

3/3 Saturday Day 142
I woke up after 8 hours ready to get shit done. I meditated, visualized, wrote my affirmations, and knocked out some work over coffee. I am fasting today. I'd like to ease that scale down a few pounds before we head to Disney next week, and I seem stuck at 185. Fasting can help.

I have worked feverishly on the Bronco and completed a task that seemed daunting before. But I stuck with it and made it happen. I also determined the best way to remove the old bearing and collar from the axle shaft and install the new ones is to take it to my buddy who is a real mechanic and let him use his hydraulic press. Should have thought of that weeks ago. Some Bronco mechanic I am.

I was thinking to myself earlier that my mind is so damn clear today and my body feels so good that I feel as good today as I did 10 years ago. Maybe better. And I just feel so in the moment and like good things are happening around me even if I don't quite see them yet. I like this place.

3/4 Sunday Day 143

Last night was awesome. We had dinner as a family again after hanging out with some friends. I just felt so open and confident and sociable. I felt like people wanted to be around me and I wanted to be around them. It helped me see how withdrawn and locked inside my own mind I had been for years and years. To the point that one of my best buddies from childhood kind of avoided me because he just did not know me anymore. But I feel like I'm back, in a way.

And something interesting happened today after church. We were on our way to eat lunch with my parents when Scarlett's mom called asking for Scarlett to be brought to her house. I was expecting to keep Scarlett today and we had not heard from her mom all weekend. We argued about it over the phone and she did what she normally does which is to get increasingly belligerent until I give in just to keep the peace. But today I gave it right back to her. Except I was calm and rational and quick thinking, albeit forceful in my tone. I drove to her house as we continued to argue on the phone so we could speak in person. It really threw her for a loop and she ended up in a cussing fit because I was not giving in to her in the least. She made a total ass of herself in front of our daughter as her melt down escalated. I remained calm and strong and pushed back without being a damn fool about it. I could see the look of utter disbelief on her face as she sat in my car in her driveway and I smiled calmly while she contorted her face into fits of rage and stupidness. In the end, we talked ourselves back to a good place and she calmed down, but I could tell it bothered her that she could not shut me down like she used to. I suggested we have a family discussion with our daughter to let her know it is okay if we argue every now and then but we still all love each other and work together, and we went inside her house and did just that.

Now, I did end up letting her spend the day with our daughter, but only because she is leaving in a couple of days for a cruise and Scarlett and I are going to Disney for spring break. So I'm getting plenty of time with my daughter. But it still felt like a little victory and the tone has been set going forward. I want us to always get along, but I don't want it to ever be at my expense.

I have the afternoon free unexpectedly and I'm buzzing with energy to go do something. Anything. I think I'll crush a killer leg workout, then work around the yard this afternoon since the weather is nice. And this evening I'll watch Narco with dad, then come home and get some writing done.

3/6 Tuesday 144

The days are just flying by. I keep waiting on drastic changes to my life - to wake up in a new world that is just awesome, but I am smart enough to know that most changes take time. And that even though some days it seems like nothing much is happening, life is so much better than it was a few months ago that you cannot even compare. Each day I awake with a sense of purpose and gratitude. I feel and look better as the weeks go by. At times I'm as horny and hard as my 15 year old self, although most days things are just normal with strong nocturnal and morning erections and a sense of confidence around women that has not been there for a long time.

Even though my bed is still empty today, I know the changes are coming. The women are coming back. First I needed to change physically. And in doing so begin to change mentally and emotionally. I have at times avoided sex for the past few years due to lack of faith in my ability to perform and being so sick I was not up to it anyway. I did manage some pretty good sex with some lovers who came along at just the right time, but it was mostly sporadic. That created a mental block towards sex that has not immediately resolved itself. But I am ready now. I feel it. I am willing to accept it may not be perfect still, but I am willing for it to be fun again. I am willing to try.

I breezed into the pharmacy yesterday to pick up my prescription strength Omega 3's, and the usual allotment of at least 3 hot women were there. A year ago I would have had my head down and got in and out as quickly as possible, trying to hide my mental and physical pain.

But yesterday I walked in like I owned the place with head held high and smile on my face. I was flirty and witty and they each wanted to engage me. My real target was Becky behind the counter, so I spoke directly to Misty and Lexi and flirted with them a bit. Becky eyed me with a smile and as I walked away she called out to me to say bye. Soon, Becky. Soon.

3/7 Wednesday Day 145
I feel good today. My mind is pretty clear and my energy is nice. I had an excellent workout this evening at the gym. If my shoulders were a bit healthier I could really kill it, but I fear I did some damage back when I was really lifting heavy several years ago. There is a good chance I'll need to get the left one cleaned up a bit someday. But for now I am careful with my range of motion.

We leave for Disney World on Friday and I am excited but nervous about that. I intend to pin late Thursday night and not pin again until I get back the following Tuesday, so I'll be off by 24 hours or so. I don't see it being a big deal but we'll see.

I am anxious for labs. I want to know my hematocrit and estradiol. It makes me nervous not knowing, but I don't go back until April 2.

3/8 Thursday Day 146
I didn't sleep much last night. I have this occasional pattern of waking up around 2 or 3. It's okay though because I still have good energy and I need to get to sleep early this evening since we are leaving so early for Disney.

When we were there last fall, I can still recall feeling shitty and so damn brain foggy I barely knew where we were. I fought suicidal thoughts the first couple of days. At damn Disneyworld! The happiest place on earth! I can remember riding the Goofy roller coaster and wishing I'd go flying out of it and die. Put me out of my misery. The thoughts subsided enough to make it an enjoyable trip, but overall I was ready to get my ass back home to the safety of my little house and my little recliner. I hope for better results this time.

3/9 Friday Day 147
We made it to Disney. I barely slept, but have managed to soldier through and keep my mood in a good place. I had a touch of anxiety on the plane, but not enough to worry me. Just mostly tired. We hit Hollywood Studios around 1PM and went straight to Rockin Roller Coaster. I can recall with shitty fondness the level of anxiety and derealization I had last year when we rode it. I forced myself to do it for my daughter, but there was nothing fun about it. This time it was fun though. I just smiled and let myself go. The rush was nice.

I did fall asleep in the damn Muppet Show and kind of freaked out when I awoke and bubbles were falling from the ceiling. I did not know what the hell was going on or where I was for a moment. Then I laughed it off. Damn Muppets.

This evening I am exhausted and my mood is a bit funky, but otherwise okay. I look forward to a good day tomorrow.

3/10 Saturday Day 148
Tough day. I slept decent. Not great, but decent. I woke up once around 2 AM and was buzzing with energy. I meditated myself back to sleep. I don't even know if I had morning wood, but I think not.

My mood continued to shift throughout the day until I was ready to get back to the room and pull the covers over my head and cry. I felt like I was not even really in existence. Like it was a bad dream I was just floating through. Then I got pissed and yelled at myself internally until I could shake off the foulness of my feelings. Depression is a bitch. At least it doesn't stay so long now. Overall the day was good. I mean, I am in Disney with my daughter and some of my best friends. My 1st world problems seem pretty damn insignificant in the grand scheme of things.

I look for better sleep tonight and a better mood tomorrow.

3/11 Sunday Day 149
Good days are here again!

I slept pretty well, got up and meditated before dawn, grabbed some coffee from the hotel snack shop, and gently woke my daughter for another fun day at Disney. Maybe I was just exhausted yesterday and the last few years have left me ill-equipped to go much without sleep.

We hit Animal Kingdom hard today and had a blast. I felt calm, confident, and generally happy. I did at times feel a punch in the gut at all the happy couples walking around while I soldiered on - a single dad with his daughter. But I tried to keep things in perspective and acknowledge how lucky I am. Besides, some of those dads looked pretty damn miserable.

3/12 Monday Day 150
My energy knows no bounds. After getting my sleep lined out, I have had good energy all day and into the evening. That is after walking miles through Disney crowds and dodging obese people on scooters. I watched as my friends wore themselves out and looked tired and haggard by the end of the days, while I was ready to keep going. I could stay a week here. Hell, a month if I could afford it.

It still amazes me how quickly my mood can shift. Lyme disease brought on these intense mood swings. Before that, I think my mood was pretty stable. Somewhere between bored and slightly optimistic. My lows are lower now, but my highs are much higher.

It's interesting to spend time here with my best buddy. Growing up, we were roughly the same size and build until high school. He hit some kind of testosterone spurt where he muscled up, developed body acne, and damn well stunk with BO for a while. And the women loved him. He was having more sex at 15 than most men in their first year of marriage. It was an amazing transformation to witness.

Now we are both over 40, and even though he is overweight from drinking thousands of Bud Lights, he is still solid as a damn oak and one of the strongest men I know. And he hasn't seen a weight room since college. He's fat though, so I can make fun of him for that.

3/13 Tuesday Day 151
I have just realized that my wood has been absent the past few mornings. So damn inconsistent. Maybe it's the Disney sweets and Disney beers. I'm on vacation so I give myself a pass.

We should have stayed longer. My head is just now getting into true vacation mode and it is time to return. I don't know why I ever take short vacations. At some point this year I'm taking a serious break. Like seven days or more. Not sure how yet, but I know I am.

I feel leaner, even with all the unhealthy Disney food. Perhaps all the walking evens things out. My left shoulder is hurting a bit from picking up my daughter. She is almost 10 but still acts like my baby. I will always hold her in my arms as long as she lets me. Shoulders be damned.

3/14 Wednesday Day 152
Already back at work. My sleep was deep last night. And I noticed on the plane I woke up gasping a few times. I really need a sleep study to check for apnea.

At times while in Disney I was worried about my blood pressure. Not sure why. I have not checked it in a while. I just felt this fullness in my veins and a pressure in my body not familiar to me. It seems to have subsided now, but it was tangible for a few days. I should get it checked.

My wood is pretty average. There is a sweet spot but I have not been able to stay on it. It is almost time to go for my checkup. I'm going to move it up to next week so I can get labs. No point in stressing about anything when I can just go find out.

Overall, I do have this sense of calmness and security that has settled in no matter what might be happening. I had not really noticed that until recently. It's like I know I can handle anything that might pop up. I like this feeling. And the feeling that many great things are on their way to me. I spent a lot of my adult life feeling most of the really great things had already happened or I had missed them altogether. That has turned around now.

3/15 Thursday Day 153

I weighed 181 at the gym. Incredible after the calories I consumed at Disney. And I feel leaner through my whole body. Pants are a bit looser. It's like the fat was stubbornly holding on for a long time, and then it released. While actually gaining a bit of muscle in my shoulders and chest. My legs need more attention. I've been wearing shorts and my calves and quads are not monstrous like I had envisioned. More like an 8th grade cheerleader. But I'll get there.

My mind has been really clear this week. And very determined to reach a level of financial freedom that allows more frequent and longer Disney trips. Among other things. I am just not meant for the daily grind of corporate America. I never was. With a clear mind and forceful feeling of determination, I am confident I can accomplish whatever I wish.

3/16 Friday Day 154

Another week in the books. I somehow forgot to set my alarm and ended up sleeping until 9 AM. It felt good though. I was exceptionally rested when I awoke. And at full attention.

I was out of needles so did not pin last night. I'm getting a bit sloppy on my schedule. I can do better on that.

So I drove to the next town over tonight to get some needles at Walgreens and had a hell of a time with the pharmacy there. Since they don't keep the needles out front, I had to request them over the counter. I asked for some 27 gauge insulin needles. She asked if I had a prescription there and I said no. So she went and got the head pharmacist. She asked again about my prescription. I told her they were for testosterone and my prescription was from my clinic in a different town, but this pharmacy was closer and I needed some syringes. She began this big lecture about buying testosterone off the street and sharing needles, like I was a heroin or meth addict. I stopped her and informed her I was on legitimate therapy and just needed some syringes. She then shifted gears and started talking about the gauge needle I really needed. She brought out some 25 gauge which would have been acceptable, but they were 3 mL and did not have small enough graduations. I told her I needed 1mL since I only use .25mL twice a week. She looked at me like I had a bird on my head. "That's a teeny tiny dose!" she exclaimed. I suppressed the urge to call her an idiot, and informed her it came out to 100 mg per week which was pretty standard. I did not even mention HCG because I did not want to melt her mind right there in front of everyone. So she want in the back and returned with some 27 gauge syringes with 1 mL tubes. Just like I asked for the first time. I smiled and thanked her and she again mentioned buying drugs off the street and said steroids are not worth it. I said, "Look, I weigh just over 180 pounds and have legs like a junior high cheerleader. Do I look like I abuse steroids?" She seemed to get the message and finally just rung up the order. What a damn adventure.

3/17 Saturday Day 155
I slept until damn near noon, but only because I stayed up drinking wine and watching a movie with my mom. May sound sad to some, but my parents are getting older and I enjoy spending time with them. They won't always be here.

After coffee and breakfast, I got some good work done on a children's affirmation book I began before I got sick. It's just about finished. Then dad and I went to town to get some yard supplies since it is spring and the weather is nice.

It's weird, but I felt very alpha walking around Lowe's and Harbour Freight Tools and wanted someone to challenge me. Like I could just whip somebody's ass if I needed to. Ha!

3/18 Sunday Day 156
Another good night of sleep. No waking up in the middle of the night wired. I got up and felt pretty damned fine and made my daughter pancakes. I had coffee and decided to fast until after noon.

My mind and vision are getting clearer by the day. At times I thought the Lyme vision issues and derealization had lifted, only to have another layer lift and get even closer to my true baseline reality. That happened a good bit this weekend. I sat yesterday afternoon at a stop sign and just marveled at how real the pavement and grass looked outside my car. Even my hands look real again - not like some rubber appendages. That's a hell of a thing to say, but that is the world of Lyme and derealization. It is why many do not make it out.

My morning wood has grown noticeably softer over the recent weeks. I wonder if my testosterone levels have gone back down as my body has adjusted to the dose. Hopefully I find out this week if I can get my appointment moved up. I read so often about men on protocols higher than mine, both in testosterone and HCG and getting marvelous results. Mine are good so far, but at times I have wondered if it is worth it. Nothing too amazing has happened yet. No women throwing their panties at me or shirts getting ripped due to my bulging muscles. Still, I'm a damn far sight from where I started.

3/19 Monday Day 157
I woke up funky this morning, but otherwise okay. I really question this apnea thing. It takes me a few minutes in the mornings to get my brain unfogged, and it could be related to oxygen. Why does TRT causes apnea?

Other than that I feel pretty okay. Had decent wood but not iron hard. Been calm and focused at work. Feel an inner drive to get some things done and be productive. This is the week to get caught up a bit before I get back on the road.

10:14 PM It was kind of a tough evening. My mood dipped for some reason and I just felt down in the dumps for a while. Then it lifted and I am okay. I wanted to hit the gym, but dad called and said he was cooking quail and I did not want to turn him down on that. I should have hit the gym then ate afterwards. I would have felt better. Now I feel bloated. I have lost 5 good pounds, but could easily put it back on if my diet is not clean. I need a good day tomorrow.

3/20 Tuesday Day 158

No wood today! I feel okay mentally - better than yesterday. But I must face reality that my wood has been steadily declining. Something is going on. No nocturnal or morning surprises. It kind of snuck up on me.

Currently I am taking .75 mg per week of anastrozole. Too much? Too little? I tried to call the clinic today to get in but it kept going to their voicemail. I'll try again tomorrow.

I will say I looked pretty lean this morning in the mirror though. Not necessarily muscular, but leaner.

And, I only slept about 6 hours last night. Had a little trouble drifting off to sleep, then woke up at 5:50 AM and that was it.

I have had good energy all day though. It is after 5 PM and I am still at work. I have been steady at it since 7 this morning. Could definitely take a nap now, but I'll hit the gym and try and get to bed early.

3/21 Wednesday Day 159

Another morning with no wood. Not sure what is going on. My sleep was decent but not great. My mind at least is very clear and focused. Mood is positive and determined.

I skipped the gym today. Had to work until after 6, and by the time I got home I was just worn out. I chilled in the recliner and let my mind go blank until Scarlett got home at 7 from church. I had great intentions of cooking a healthy meal tonight, but looks like it is not happening. Maybe tomorrow night.

3/22 Thursday Day 160

No wood. Mind clear. Sleep was fitful. Need a better day. What's happening to me?

3/23 Friday Day 161

We have wood! I did my pin last night, but I am officially out of HCG. I slept like a baby and woke up at 6 AM ready to drive nails. Is there a connection or just a coincidence? I also have not drank any wine this week. Maybe that is a larger contributor. I have an appointment on Monday to get my bloods done and pick up some more HCG. I'll adjust based on that.

I missed the gym again last night. My ex insisted we go as a family to shop for birthday invitations and decorations for our daughter. I had to say yes. We ended up eating Chinese buffet afterwards, so not only did I miss gym this week I topped it off with a shitty meal. I'll never see those abs with weeks like this!

But I know I'll get back on track. I do fear that I have a hernia on my right side. I think it has been there for a while and they missed it when they repaired the one on the left. It hurts when I turn or bend over, and I can feel it when I strain. If I have it repaired I'll go the laparoscopic route - no more mesh. It could possibly be pulling my right nut up high since the left one hangs a good bit lower and freer. So many damn things to look into. When is the last time I was completely healthy?

My mind has been wonderful this week though. Very clear and focused and lots of great ideas flowing through me. I made good progress on some writing projects I have going which is always fulfilling. I watch my old buddy Matthew Lewis on Facebook hopping from one vacation to the next after his success with a board game he invented, and I know it will be me on there someday with something I have created. Not necessarily travelling the world drinking beer and wine like he is, but doing what I want with my time instead of what a corporation tells me to. It's coming. Maybe. I need a break from this monotony. Something needs to give, and soon. What does a vagina look like? I forget. I'm taking a break from journaling. I write the same shit everyday and nothing much changes. Up then down. Down then up. Shit, I need a break.

BLUE SKIES SHINING ON ME

6/11/18 Monday
My break paid off. I needed to stop creating the same reality over and over. I needed a new script for this thing called life. I had to break the monotony of journaling about the same shit day in day out.

I feel great. I have an erection that could smash boards every morning. I had amazing sex only a couple weekends ago, and look forward to some more this coming weekend.

My mind is crystal clear most days.

I am stronger.

Determined and focused.

I have elevated myself in my current job even as I seek other ventures.

During social gatherings I engage rather than hang out in the shadows.

I had a party at my house Friday night and it was awesome.

I pray and meditate each morning, and lift 3 times per week.

Life is pretty damn good right now.

What else has changed since I took a break?

Still actively working to get estrogen in check. It gets high, then it gets low. I am extremely sensitive to Arimidex, but using Calcium D-Glucarate alone is not enough. My next move is to increase my injection frequency to EOD. Currently I am still on 100 mg 2x week, along with 250 ml of HCG 2x week.

I have some back acne but it's not terrible. Just enough to annoy the hell out of me.

And even though my diet has been 50% good and 50% shit, my body composition is pretty nice. Less than 20% body fat while drinking a glass of wine 2-3 times per week and eating out often with my work travel. I went to a conference last week and had huge corporate dinners each night. Drinks, appetizers, dessert. I lost a pound.

But I can do better. With just a little bit of diet effort I could be freaking ripped right now. I don't need wine every night. It's not *that* good for my heart. It's amazing how poor my diet has been while still maintaining a decent body. But it's hard when I travel so much for work.

My sleep is great - better than it's been in years. Even if I only get 5-6 hours I have energy all day. And I can sleep a good 8 when it's available and get up ready to kick some ass. I never did get that sleep study, but if I avoid sleeping flat on my back I don't seem to snore that bad. Sleeping on my side works just fine.

I've felt so good that I have spent a considerable amount of time just taking in certain moments. Watching bees on flowers, petting my dog, watching my daughter sleep. Just living in the bliss of life. No pressure to be something else or somewhere else. Just contentment. Just being.

It seems all of my adult life I felt I had to get to someplace to be happy. To accomplish certain things. To achieve. Now I feel perfectly content in the moment, while fanning the flames of desire to do great things.

I've written a considerable amount in my novel. I have published some good blog posts. I am working on other business ventures. Pushing profitability on my rental properties. Keeping things moving while staying grounded in the moments.

But it's not perfect. I desire more sex. I look for sexual opportunities in my small town only to continue to find limited availability. I am on 2 internet dating sites but no matches worth exploring so far. I have considered pursuing a few ladies who do not meet my current standards in the name of increased sexual activity, but I am not that desperate yet. I still believe I can re-establish a fine sex life with acceptable partners without sacrificing personal preferences. But how long I hold to my principles remains to be seen.

I leave for vacation tomorrow. A week of cold beer on the beach just watching the waves crash in. I need the downtime. I get so much done in a 16 hour day now compared to a few months ago it is mind boggling, but I still have a breaking point for stress. I do not intend to find out what that is.

I will continue to chronicle this journey. I felt bad taking so much time off from my journal, but I needed to quit repeating the same thing day in and day out. I was creating the same reality over and over. It is what it is. And it is getting better.

6/17 Sunday
It's father's day. We've been on the beach since Tuesday. I have felt solid and in a good mood all week. It's actually been weird to be here and just live day to day - not trapped inside my own head. Sometimes I get a little bit weirded out like I can no longer relate to the neurotic and fearful man I have been these past few years. I just live man. I feel like The Dude.

It's by no means perfect. I am by no means perfect. I ogled teen girls in bikinis all week at the beach, and I'll soon by 43. I started to feel guilty about that, then I let my mind wander into the evolution of mankind and how for thousands of years it would have been perfectly acceptable for me to take one of those girls. Now it is considered a felony. Well, they mostly appeared to be around 18 so not a felony but definitely frowned upon. So I feel no guilt.

I also noticed that I saw hundreds of women this week and maybe one my age that looked decent in a swimsuit. Perhaps it is just this part of the country and characteristic of who vacations at the Gulf of Mexico, but damnit man. I expected more than that. I did see plenty of dudes who keep in shape and several who have to be supplementing more than a just a little bit.

I myself felt pretty muscular out there in spite of my poor diet and frequent drinking. And each day I seem to wake up leaner no matter how crappy I eat the day before.

And here is some interesting trivia. The saga of my estrogen may be solved, at least for now. I was positive it was creeping up on me since I had dropped the AI after bottoming out at 9. I had blood drawn Tuesday before I left to come down here, and checked my results online yesterday. My total T was around 900, and my estrogen was 25. Damn near perfect! I have been taking Calcium d-Glucarate and I guess it holds the line. Hell that tells me that I was probably still low for weeks and just now recovered from the AI. I am that damn sensitive to it! Oh well. I had pinned the day before so I am curious about my T being 900. Is that a peak or close to it? I think maybe not peak but certainly not valley. Seems like a good number and I feel pretty good, so no adjustments necessary. And my hematocrit was 42! That's a great number.

I'll admit, I do still worry about my long-term heart health. The next numbers to get are my lipid profile. If it is not better then I'll take a low level statin as much as I don't want to do it. I just can't keep going with low HDL and high LDL. I'll stress about it daily and just generate unwanted anxiety. But maybe all the fish oil and omegas are helping. Not sure the red yeast rice does much but I'm still taking it.

Overall I like where I am. My next quest is to sharpen my focus on a project I've had in my mind for months. For years I have struggled to focus on accomplishing goals, even in my prime. Maybe it was hormones; maybe it was laziness and lack of discipline. Either way I feel mentally strong enough now to get some shit done in dramatic fashion, and I don't give a shit what anyone else thinks of me. So I will daily scribe about my progress, then move onto the next one.

That is exactly what I am willing to do.

6/19 Tuesday
Had sex last night. And again this morning. Last night it was over too quickly, but this morning was a good session. I forgot how much I enjoyed it. Just being in the moment. Not too caught up with it being perfect, just letting go and giving it my all. It's a beautiful fucking thing.

My body continues to look leaner despite my poor diet. What could I do with a spot on diet, absence of alcohol, and intense workout routine? Shit.

I am at the Beau Rivage casino in Biloxi, MS about to attend an OSHA VPP conference. Not the most exciting stuff, but it's necessary right now for what I do. Of course I want to write. To create and work from my computer wherever I choose to be. I thought that was just a dream for a while, but damn if I don't have the confidence that I can make it happen now.

Lots of things are slowly coming together. Can I make them happen faster? Perhaps. But I like where I am. No depression. No anxiety. No joint pain. Performance anxiety fading away. Shyness not an issue and inner dialogue positive. It's a good time to be me. Only been a few times in my life have I said those words.

6/25 Monday
I'm about to jump into a huge opportunity at work. I have essentially been offered a plant manager's job at the factory I once worked at. Unfreaking-believable. No way would I have had the courage to take such a job in the past. I would have been too damn worried about having all the men on the factory floor like me and approve of me. I would have been tentative and timid and they would have eaten me for breakfast every day. Not after the journey I've been on these past few years. I know I can do this damn job. So I reached out to the hiring manager and threw my hat in the ring. I think he was as surprised as I was. I figured fuck it and I just took a chance. Now look what is happening!

Since I last had my blood checked a few weeks ago, my morning erections seem to be getting fuller. I like that and they are very nice to wake up to.

My weight seems stuck at 181. It's been there for a while now. No matter how much or how crappy I eat, my body composition stays pretty decent and my weight stays stable. Interesting. At 175 I'd have pretty good definition right now, but here I am at 181. It's not a bad place.

My sleep is good, although I still want that sleep study. Probably a little apnea. Better safe than sorry.

7/2 Monday
I have felt better than ever this past week. I stopped taking the iodine supplement and I think it helped. I suppose I bought into the online hype and thought I needed super high levels of iodine to function, but it appears I feel just fine on normal levels I get through food and whatever is in my multivitamin. The best thing that has helped me feel good is eating breakfast every day. I know I can lean down pretty easily when I intermittent fast, but it leaves me feeling cold and my body feels like it does not get good blood flow. I think it was even affecting my erections because they are stronger than ever now. I wake up at night and first thing in the morning with a boner so hard a damn cat couldn't scratch it. It's like I'm 18 again. I feel I'm wielding a lightsaber, or a meat saber, everywhere I go – and pussy best beware.

I slept 7 solid hours last night as usual and woke up ready to get shit done. It's a good feeling to be focused and on point. Over the weekend I played in a golf tournament and where in the past I have been content to sit in the cart and stay quiet and observe others get excited, I was more of the team cheerleader and coach this year and we won our flight. I kept our energy high and positive and we played some of our best golf over two days. It was a hoot!

7/5 Thursday
My sleep was deep last night but not enough. The past few nights I've been staying up until midnight or later instead of getting to bed a decent hour.

I am pushing the limits of how effective I can be on reduced sleep. Still pretty damn effective!

My back and chest are breaking out again. Not pretty. Maybe it's the Mississippi heat and the sweat, or maybe my estrogen is just fluctuating. I have not taken any AI in a couple of weeks now, and even then it was only 1/8 of a mg. Mentally I have felt a little cloudy but my mood has been nice. Just kind of floating along. It would be so helpful to have a simple at home monitor for estrogen - the way diabetics have for blood sugar. I'm not saying check it every day, but at least weekly until everything is really dialed in.

I awoke around 2AM with a boner so hard I thought it might burst. I mean it was like steel pipe hard. Those things just keep getting better and better. I like it.

So where do I go from here? The days keep getting better. I have enjoyed some nice sex. I managed to take a quantum leap in my career. I am stronger than I have ever been. Lyme disease can kiss my ass. Life is good. Maybe I'll have to stick myself with a needle twice a week until I am a wrinkly old man, but I'll be a muscular wrinkly old man still having sex and kicking ass at life. It is a small price to pay. I am willing to pay it.

CONCLUSION

I debated on sharing this journal. It's mostly just me going on and on about trying to improve my life. Who would want to read that? I am positive most people have their shit together and are not interested in one man's struggle to find some sense of joy and peace in his daily routine. But for those who don't, maybe someone will get something out of this.

Rereading the entries of my journey into testosterone replacement therapy, it really was a kick in the gut to realize that even as some things got better I stayed stuck in old patterns way too long. I had to take a step back from what was normal, take some different actions, and make a move in my life. Nothing really changed until I did.

I will say, however, that I would likely still be in those same old patterns if not for TRT. It may not have forced any different decisions by itself, but it was certainly the catalyst that helped me make needed changes.

One of the biggest differences I noticed in my mindset was the absolute indifference to what others thought of me. I never realized before how much other people's opinion limited my thoughts and actions. The confidence I gained from having high T levels - that edge I developed from feeling "on" most of the time - it obliterated my ability to give a shit what other people think. No way would I have stepped into the job I have now before. Ever. There is simply too much pressure and too much criticism from too many people. But step into it I did, and what a wonderful experience that has been to go from a one man show to leading men on a daily basis. TRT gifted that to me.

Sex was a tricky problem to solve. I had a fairly normal sex life up until I got sick with Lyme disease. That hell that is borne from a tick upset my bodily functions so much that having sex was the least of my worries. But I did try a few times even during my sickest days to enjoy a romp with some willing women, and it just wasn't happening. It struck a serious blow to my confidence. So much so that even after I was better and even after I was sailing on the high seas of TRT I was hesitant to initiate a sexual encounter. It just took some time. And it was worth the wait. Sex was just as much fun as it always has been. I will say the desire is a little deeper now. Something similar to what I remember from my teens and early 20's with that longing in my loins. It is a good feeling. I also remembered that sex does not have to be perfect. It is not a porno. It is made for our enjoyment and there does not have to be any added pressure to it.

My social life is an interesting thing to behold now. Even before I got sick, I was not the most social person. I was not necessarily uncomfortable in social situations, but unless the booze was flowing I tended to hang back and mostly keep to myself. I preferred a night at home or with a small group of friends rather than a big crowd. And there was never anything really wrong with that. But there has definitely been a shift in that department. I take some enjoyment in being a part of a large crowd now, and even more than that I want them to hear what I have to say. Not from the perspective that I need to dominate like some alpha male, but from a need for socialization that I did not feel before. I think part of it stems from not caring if others judge me. It allows me to feel more comfortable sharing myself with people. But a part of it also grows from a need to share whatever I have to offer with others. Not just keep it to myself. To be a part of something bigger than my own individual thoughts. That is the best way I know to describe it.

Things that still worry me are my heart health. My lipid panel without a doubt took a turn for the worse once I began TRT. I am taking statins now to manage that, but I am not excited about it. The research is fuzzy. The TRT community online is adamant there is no evidence that testosterone therapy can cause heart issues. Statements like "testosterone is heart protective" are commonly thrown around as fact. The same for estrogen. "It's better to be a little high than a little low" has become adopted certitude. What is the truth? Much more research needs to be done. What I do know is that high LDL and low HDL levels are a recipe for disaster. There is not much to question about that.

Hematocrit is something to watch, but apparently I was naturally a bit low before I started so now my levels stay in a good place. That is comforting. Part of me wants to know why I was a little low, but not all numbers can be in the perfect range. It is enough for now that I am not at risk.

My blood pressure rose some initially, but that was not necessarily a bad thing. It dropped too low when I was really sick. It was common to collapse into a clinic observation room and see numbers like 90/60, with the nurse telling me I must be a marathon runner. It hurt too much to laugh at the time. After climbing up to a little on the high side, it now rests mostly in the normal range. That 120/80 golden ratio. That's good.

The wrestling match with estrogen may never end, but the fluctuations are much less than before. I have it mostly managed with Calcium D-Glucarate, but I know after a while just the tiniest bit of an AI is necessary to dial it back down. I can mostly go by feel at this point, but I still long for the day a simple at home test comes out.

As for pinning, it's a breeze. I have no issues traveling with my kit, and if I skip a dose of HCG I don't even notice. I move the injection sites around so I have no scar tissue, and I order my syringes off of Amazon so I don't have to argue with the idiots at the pharmacy about what gauge I need and the dangers of steroid abuse.

This is a life that millions of men have chosen, or in many cases this life has chosen them. In the coming years TRT will be pretty commonplace. More and more men will wake up to the benefits of having optimized hormones, and the stigma will continue to drop. I have no doubts about that. Will I continue on my path? Maybe. Part of me really needs to know how my body can function free and clear of Lyme disease. Part of me needs to know if I can be natural again. But if this is my fate, so be it. It's a good life.

www.ingramcontent.com/pod-product-compliance
Lightning Source LLC
Chambersburg PA
CBHW021340290326
41933CB00037B/311